Injury Prevention and Care in Artistic Sports

Henrique Jones • Angelina Lukaszenko
Editors

Injury Prevention and Care in Artistic Sports

Springer

European Society of Sports Traumatology, Knee Surgery & Arthroscopy
ESSKA

Editors
Henrique Jones
Hospital da Luz, Setúbal Orthopedic
Surgery and Sports Medicine
Montijo Orthopedic Sports Med Clinic
Setubal, Portugal

Angelina Lukaszenko
Abu Dhabi, UAE

ISBN 978-3-032-18104-6 ISBN 978-3-032-18105-3 (eBook)
https://doi.org/10.1007/978-3-032-18105-3

Cover images: The photos reproduced on the book cover are licensed from Getty Images (from left to right):

Saro17 / E+ Collection via Getty Images; Alexandr Dubynin / Moment Collection via Getty Images; Artur Didyk / iStock / Getty Images Plus via Getty Images; Serhii Prystupa / Moment Collection via Getty Images; German-skydiver / iStock / Getty Images Plus via Getty Images

This Springer imprint is published by the registered company Springer Nature Switzerland AG
The registered company address is: Gewerbestrasse 11, 6330 Cham, Switzerland

If disposing of this product, please recycle the paper.

Contents

1 Equestrian Sport

Angelina Lukaszenko

1.1 Introduction

Equestrian sport is one of the most popular sport nowadays around the world. Dealing with an animal that is able to think, react, and breathe on its own creates "magic" that is able to put a spell on almost everyone who really tries to tame the horse (Fig. 1.1). Since ancient times, horses were parts of myths and legends and never presented as a weak and dependable creature. Being with a horse give people ability to feel free and magnificent.

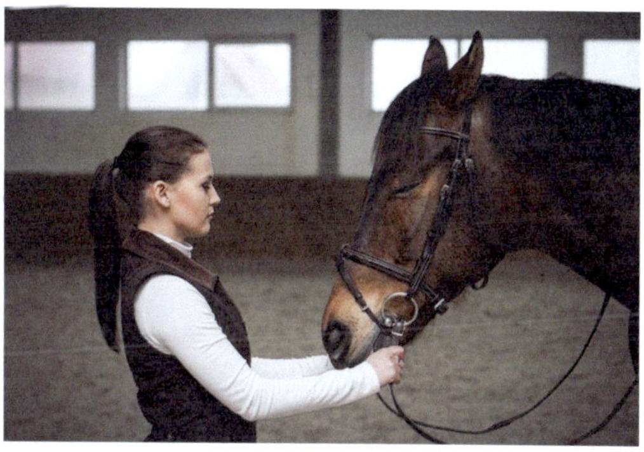

Fig. 1.1 Human and horse can understand each other by nonverbal language

A. Lukaszenko (✉)
Abu Dhabi, UAE

H. Jones, A. Lukaszenko (eds.), *Injury Prevention and Care in Artistic Sports*,
https://doi.org/10.1007/978-3-032-18105-3_1

1.2 History and Tradition in Most Important Equestrian Discipline

Over the years, the equestrian sport evolved, creating specific disciplines. Those disciplines were named and categorized according to the International Equestrian Federation (FEI):

(a) Show jumping: a strategic ride where horse and rider pass the parkour (8–11 obstacles) in as short time as possible without any fouls (Fig. 1.2). Horse and rider could compete on time, amount of mistakes, or quality of riding style. Nevertheless, good mathematical precision and strategic mind can be keys to success. A standard parkour consists of 11 obstacles with different shapes and length. Some obstacles can be filled by water, where some can be shaped in waves. One of the most spectacular shows with obstacles is a music and speed show, where horse and rider finish the parkour as fast as possible all while surrounded by loud, energetic music. The biggest challenge for balance, coordination, and precision is the high jump competition. Two meters and above high of an obstacle can cause fear to a lot of riders, but those who can jump it are usually the most balanced athletes (together with the horse as a partner).

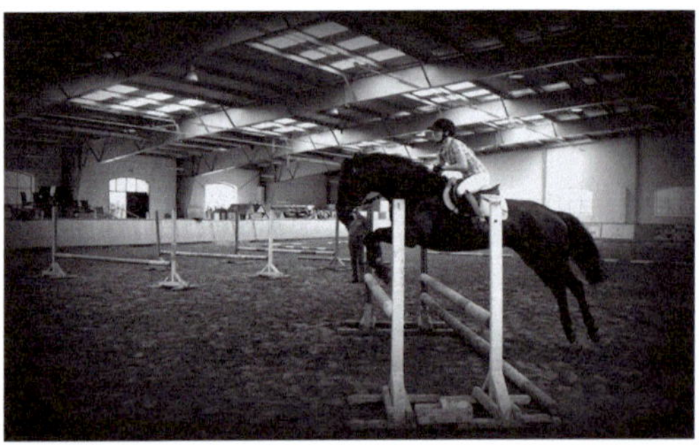

Fig. 1.2 Jumping training

(b) Dressage (Fig. 1.3a) and para-dressage: high-skilled horse "art" where horse and rider demonstrate long/short steps, pirouettes, stepping in one place and controlled gallop in a full balance. "Horse dancing" is performed usually with music (on the advanced levels) and can give an impression of an easy and comfortable riding in full balance and understanding with the horse, but the truth is that this kind of communication with an animal requires a lot of practice, balance, and knowledge of the rider's own body. To be able to separately using hands, wrists, pelvic, knees and foot during the "pirouette "in gallop.

(c) Eventing: where a couple rider and a horse compete in a three-round competition: cross-country, dressage, and show jumping.

(d) Driving (Fig. 1.3b) and para-driving: includes carriage driving by one, two, four, or even six horses. Reminding XVII centuries carriages and long journeys through forests and narrow roads of small cities. Nowadays competitions have even more advantages then in previous centuries daily living traveling.

(e) Endurance: long-distance riding in different environments like desert or forest. It looks like one of the most easiest equestrian disciplines, but it's not. It requires a lot of stamina and endurance from both the rider and the horse.

(f) Vaulting: a combination of gymnastic skills and horse riding.

(g) Raining: a Western type of riding where the rider has to complete challenges based on loops, stops, and spins in a short period of time without abusing the animal.

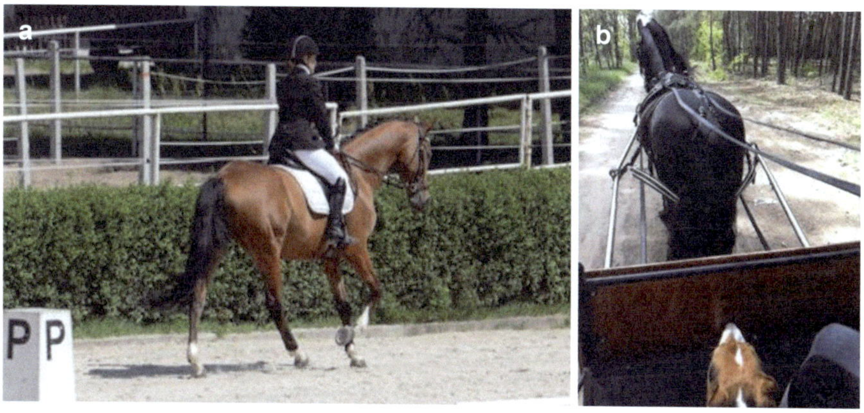

Fig. 1.3 (**a**) Dressage exhibition. (**b**) Driving

Understanding the pure connection with an animal whose power is 100% bigger than human makes horse riding one of the most beautiful but dangerous sports. Injuries and their consequence can have significant effect on the athlete. In this chapter, we will try to show how important good coordination, understanding of your own body, warming up before training, adequate treatment, and proper physiotherapy plan are. By understanding the primary mechanisms of injury, we can design specialized prevention programs for both amateurs or professional riders in all age groups. Prevention programs should focus on choosing better equipment and well-trained animals and putting more attention on warming-up as part of training. Basically we cannot say that this sport is different than any other sport there is.

1.3 Epidemiology of Injuries

Like every sport, horse riding requires a team of professionals to help the rider along the way, which includes a physician, physiotherapist, coach, and psychologist. Animals are unpredictable, and even a well-trained horse can break the bond between its human. Injuries differ between amateur and professional riders. The most frequent injuries involve the head (Table 1.1) and neck, which can lead to skull traumas, concussion, brain hematoma, bone fractures, and muscles ruptures (Table 1.2).

Table 1.1 Head injuries profile

Injury classification	
Severity	Brain injury
Minor	Concussion but awake
Moderate	Concussion with moderate consciousness
Serious	Cerebral contusion
Severe	Subdural hematoma
Critical	Specific brain mass injury
Unsurvivable	Laceration of brain stem

1.4 An Example of a Prevention Plan

Like in every sport, warming up and stretching after every ride can prevent injuries, especially if we are talking about muscle and ligament injuries. Discussed below is a simple gym-training plan for riders (Figs. 1.4, 1.5, 1.6, 1.7, and 1.8).

Table 1.2 Common injuries

		Injuries				Helmets usage	
		Concussion/ head injury	Hemorrage/ contusion/ laceration/sprain	Death	Disability	Helmets	Helmetless
Kraus [1]	155 (23%) had at least one fracture of the skull or facial bones	483 children	81 children	21	11	-	
Christoph et al. [2]	75/100 000- children	10	5	2-basiliar skull fracture		20	10
Chitnavis et al. [3]	177 children/adults	140	70	1		130	47
DeVivo [4]	75 (9 children)	33	42	5		10	
Petridou et al. [5]	244	47	200				
Thomas [6]	102 904	11 502	32 293				
Short et al. [7]	312	7,2				28 children	
Meredith et al. [8]	7815 (horse related injuries)	562	6677			1872	1680

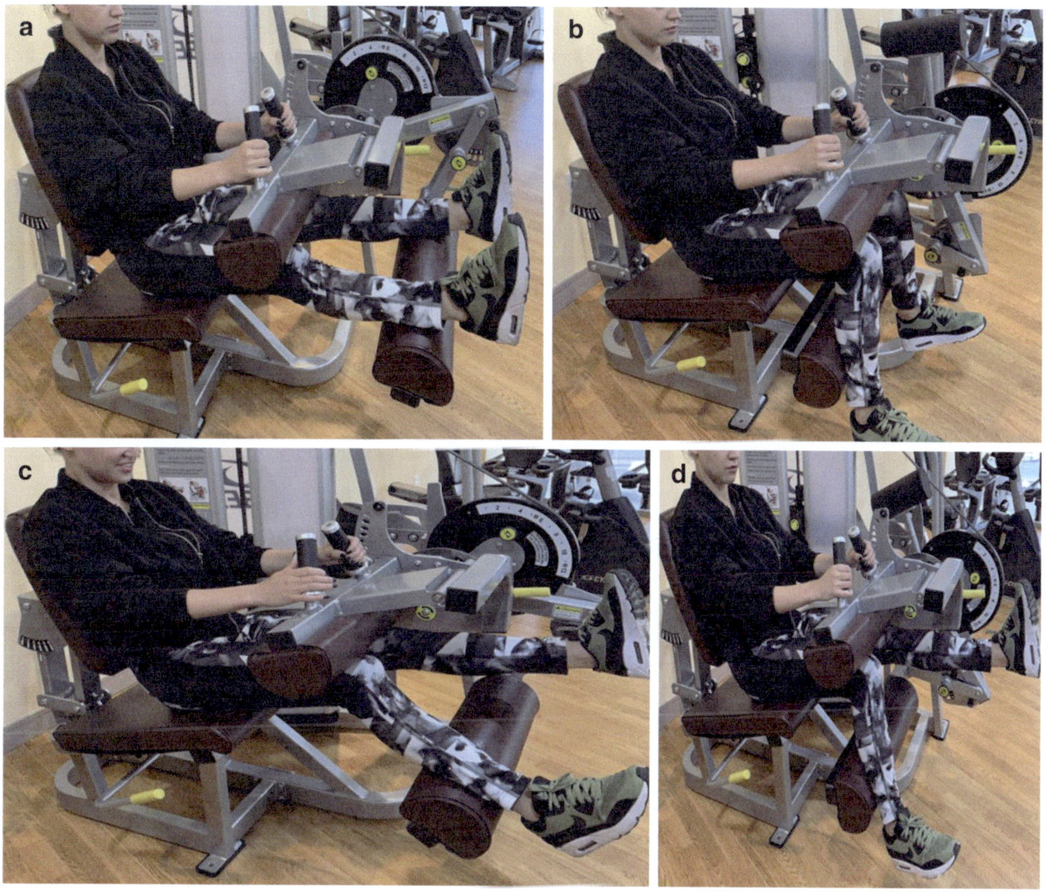

Fig. 1.4 Example of Gym- training exercise: (**a**, **b**, **c** and **d**) Leg extension and coordination

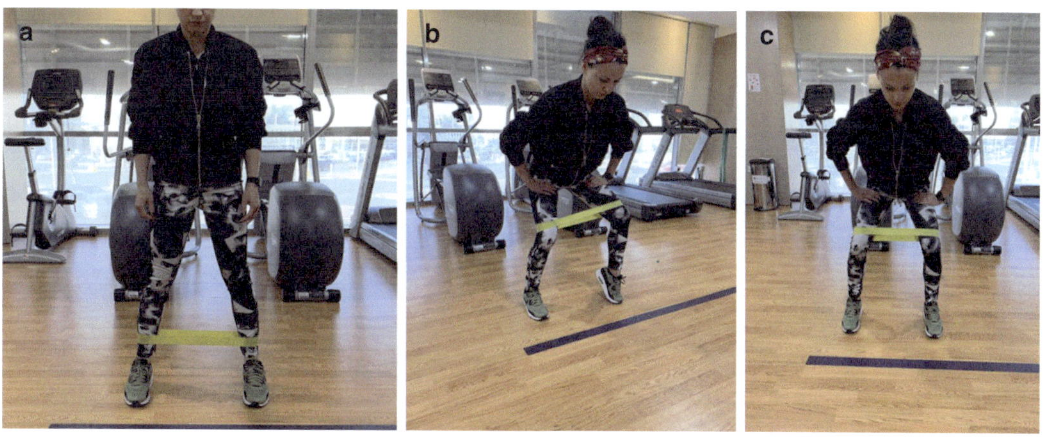

Fig. 1.5 (**a**, **b**, **c**) Leg curl work

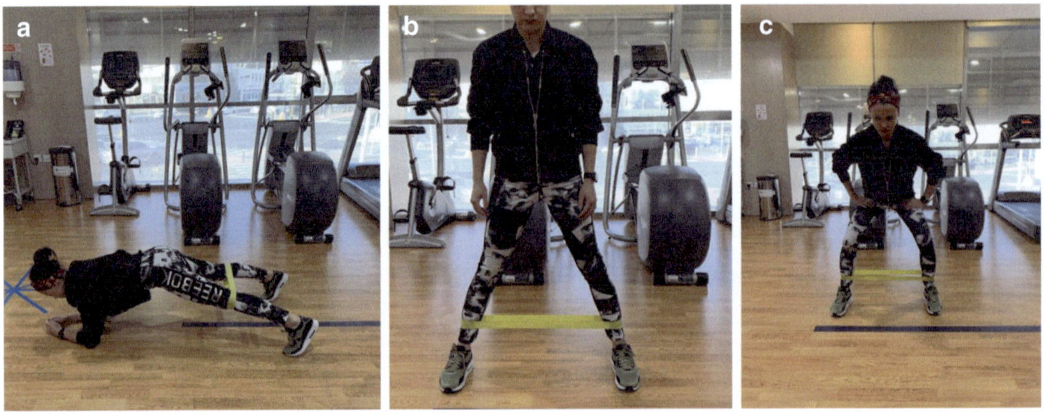

Fig. 1.6 Side walk gluteus exercises: (**a**) straight legs horizontal position, (**b**) straight legs vertical position and C squat position

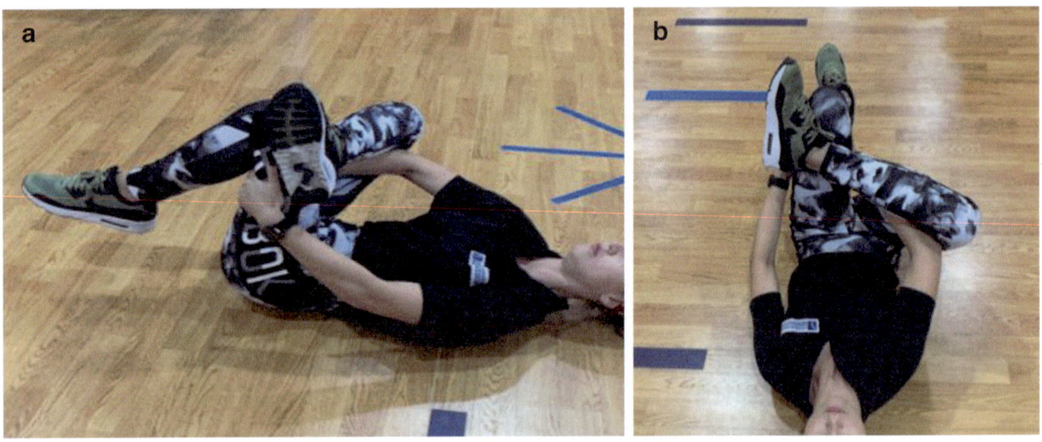

Fig. 1.7 Stretching exercises for (**a**) hip flexors and (**b**) abductors muscles

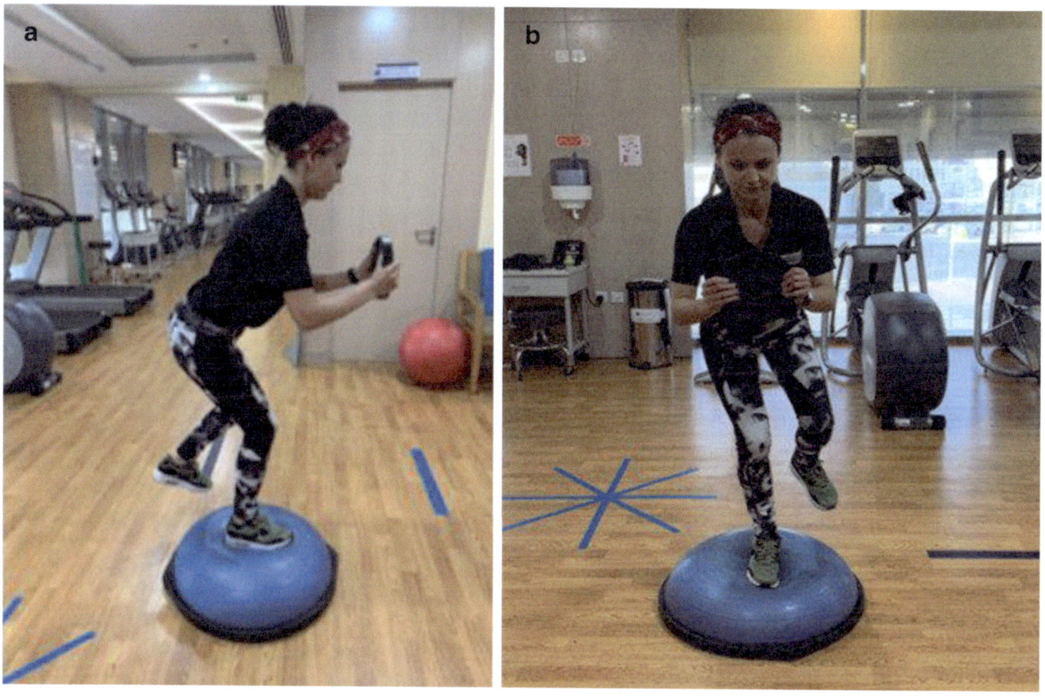

Fig. 1.8 (**a**) and (**b**) Stability, balance and proprioception exercises

Leg curl is an exercise that strengthens the hamstring muscles on the back of the thigh by bending the knee against resistance. It is performed by using each leg separatcly or together (Fig. 1.5).

Side walking with rubber has the goal of activating gluteus muscles. It is performed with straight legs or in a squat position (Fig. 1.6).

Stretching is also an important exercise that requires putting a body part in a certain position to lengthen and elongate the muscle or muscle group, thus enhancing its flexibility and elasticity (Fig. 1.7).

Core stability, balance, and proprioception relate to your inner core muscles. These muscles stabilize your spine. Core strength relates to the outer core muscles and is developed to help you move around, better preparing the body to exercise (Fig. 1.8).

1.5 Evaluation Plan

The equestrian sport is no different than any other sports regarding fitness goals and performance. Like every player, the rider should pass the evaluation process as requirement for the riding classes. Proper assessment should be made by a team of professionals toward structure of muscle, tendons, and bones, as well as biomechanics of joints and quality of movement. Psychological ability of the rider is also a vital part of the assessment. Proper evaluation should consider:

- Past injury.
- Hour spending on riding.
- Events during the season.
- Riding discipline preferences.
- Additional training outside stable premises like in the gym, Pilates, etc.
- Range of motion of joints.
- BMI.
- Length of the limbs.
- Spine problems and back pain.
- Psychological ability.
- Body parameters.

Team consisting with physicians, physiotherapist, coach, and parents should understand the specific work environment of a rider and consequences that this sport brings with it.

1.6 Proper Equipment

Like in every sport, essential equipment is critical for safety during riding lessons. Helmets (Fig. 1.9a) work provide head protection for the rider especially during height-based sports like eventing, show jumping, and endurance. Prior to mounting or even when on ground, the rider should wear a helmet, as studies show that most skull fractures happen due to being kicked by a horse during pre-ride work. In the world exists evidence which can prove that even if you have a helmet it would not protect you from brain injury or concussion- that is why more research are needed in this field.

Protective stirrups are used to protect the rider from being trapped in the saddle in case of falls. They are especially designed with a release mechanism that opens, allowing the rider's foot to let loose on the ground preventing from being pulled on the ground behind the animal, for example, when a horse gains a speed of almost 100 km/h, causing a lot of serious injuries.

Vests nowadays exist with airbag protection. All vests should be well fitted to the rider to better protect bones like collarbone, scapula, or spine from fractures during falls (Fig. 1.9b).

Reins should not be too long or too short for the to provide soft contact with the horse's mouth. The rider is also not advised to tighten the reins

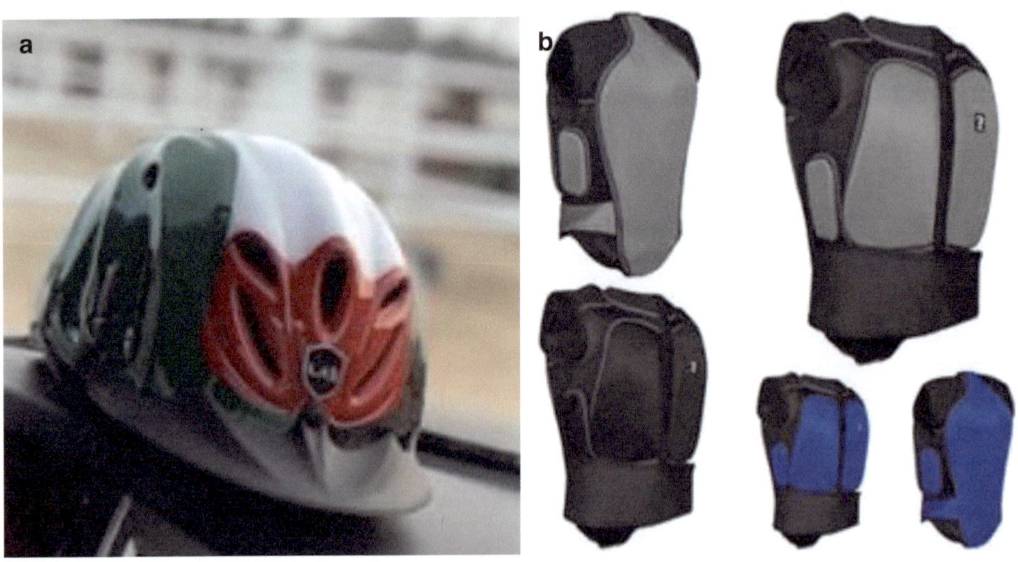

Fig. 1.9 (**a**) Helmet (**b**) Back prevention device

around their fingers or wrists as it has dangerous consequences.

The saddle should be safe for the rider and the horse's back. Too big a saddle can cause unstable position during the ride, which can cause bumping movements and pain on the horse's back, causing the rider to feel very "loose" and muscle-twitch to protection mode. Persistent muscle twitching can cause rider's deep muscles to become less elastic, which can lead to shortness in movement and misunderstanding in terms of signals the rider can send to the animal.

1.7 The Reality of Riding Traumatology

Injuries in equestrian sports have been recognized since the existence of the sport itself, and there have been published studies about them, including some pediatric injuries. Since 1987, major injuries are related to head trauma, with the worst consequences being neurological dysfunctions and death. Of the 688 children who were admitted to a hospital in the study of Kraus et al., 155 (23%) had at least 1 fracture of the skull or facial bones, with one child dying in the OR due to skull fracture and traumatic brain injury. Most of the non-neurological injuries are related to bone fractures, dislocations or muscle sprain, strain or bruising, and abrasions. Most of the injuries are related to a specific body part that includes the hands and wrists (rolling the rains around the fingers), ankles, joints (consequences of a non-safe stirrups and being trapped in the saddle), clavicle, bone (usually happens when the rider is thrown from the horse or simply falls down from the saddle), facial bones, and abdominal soft tissues (consequences of a horse kick). Only 5% of people who ride horses professionally or on an amateur level are using full protective equipment, including ground work and mounting.

1.8 Summary

The equestrian sport is considered more dangerous than other sports such as soccer, ice hockey, motorcycle, skiing, automobile racing, football, and rugby, because the rider depends on a largely unpredictable animal capable of speeds of up to 70 kph, with a weight of 1500 pounds and kicking force of up to 1 ton. Although horse riding–related injuries have been decreasing by about 40% for 20 years, they still result in a significant number of injuries. Loder et al. detected more 5033 equestrian-related injuries in the US National Trauma Data Bank between 2002 and 2004, with the most significant being head/neck trauma accounting for 23.8%, the latter increasing the risk of concussion and severe neurological disabilities.

Bibliography

1. Kraus JF, McArthur DL, Silberman TA. Epidemiology of mild brain injury. InSeminars Neurol. 1994;01;1–7. © 1994 by Thieme Medical Publishers, Inc.
2. Christoph RA, Rodgers BM, Bond G. Weston M. Pediatric equestrian injuries: assessing the impact of helmet use: Pediatrics. 1995;95:487–489. J Emerg Med. 1995;13(6):870–1.
3. Chitnavis JP, Gibbons CL, Hirigoyen M, Parry JL, Simpson AH. Accidents with horses: what has changed in 20 years?. Injury. 1996;27(2):103–5.
4. DeVivo MJ. Head neck injuries in industries. Front Head Neck Trauma Clin Biomech. 1998;21:92.
5. Petridou E, Kedikoglou S, Belechri M, Ntouvelis E, Dessypris N, Trichopoulos D. The mosaic of equestrian-related injuries in Greece. J Trauma Acute Care Surg. 2004;56(3):643–7.
6. Thomas KE, Annest JL, Gilchrist J, Bixby-Hammett DM. Non-fatal horse related injuries treated in emergency departments in the United States, 2001–2003. Br J Sports Med. 2006;40(7):619–26.
7. Short SS, Fenton SJ, Scaife ER, Bucher BT. Helmet under-utilization by children during equestrian events is associated with increased traumatic brain injury. J Pediatr Surg. 2018;53(3):545–7.
8. Meredith L, Ekman R, Thomson R. Horse-related incidents and factors for predicting injuries to the head. BMJ Open Sport Exer Med. 2018;13:4(1).

2 Circus

Michael R. Carmont

2.1 Introduction

Roll up, roll up, welcome to the Circus, the Greatest Show on Earth: Circus Injuries.

Circus performers demonstrate strength, range of movement and coordination in both acrobatic and non-acrobatic elements. They now have training programmes and performances comparable to artistic and rhythmic gymnastics and as a result have comparable injury incidence. This chapter provides a review of injuries sustained during this form of performance art. This chapter will be of use to those performing research on circus injuries and physiotherapists approached by circus performers.

2.2 History of Circus

The term "circus" relates to the word "circle" relating to a round form like a circle. In ancient Rome, charioteers would race in the Circus Maximus in a valley between the Palatine and Aventine hills. This distinguishes the Circus Maximus from the Coliseum, the site of gladiatorial combat and fights to the death.

Modern circus has been defined as a company of performers who put on a diverse entertainment show that may include clowns, acrobats, trained animals, trapeze acts, musicians, dancers, hopers, tightrope walkers, jugglers, magicians, unicyclists and stunt-oriented artists.

An ex-cavalry officer, Philip Astley is considered to be the founder of the modern circus that performs tricks and stunts whilst riding a horse south of the River Thames in London. This gives rise to the circus ring of approximately 13 m in diameter, the size of the turning circle of a horse at a canter. The modern circus consists of skilled acts choreographed by a ring master.

Arguably the greatest showman, Phineas Barnum featured may acts which some would consider to be a freak show exhibiting dwarfs and people with facial disfigurements and genetic and endocrine abnormalities.

This show series reached an end and progressed to shows featuring caged lions, tigers, bears and elephants. In some circuses, these animals were housed in very poor conditions and occasionally turned on their ring masters, who may have been termed lion tamers. These animals had the chance to exact revenge on their tormentors contrasting with other cultural activities.

The term "contemporary circus" introduces an increase in the number of acrobatic and artistic acts with a reduction in animal performances. In 1919, Lenin described the circus as the people's art form leading to the state university having classes in circus and a variety of other acts, with

M. R. Carmont (✉)
The Department of Trauma & Orthopaedic Surgery, Princess Royal Hospital, Shrewsbury & Telford Hospital NHS Trust, Shropshire, UK

H. Jones, A. Lukaszenko (eds.), *Injury Prevention and Care in Artistic Sports*,
https://doi.org/10.1007/978-3-032-18105-3_2

the Moscow Circus School being founded in the 1920s. Here, children and adolescents were taught almost in parallel with those involved in the artistic gymnastics programme.

2.3 Different Skills of the Same Sport

Participation in contemporary circus requires a high degree of acrobatic, athletic and aesthetic ability. Intense physical training is involved with an extreme range of movement and yet high physical loads often at maximum strength (Fig. 2.1). Loads are suddenly applied in compression and distraction. Additionally loads may be applied when the participant is standing on the ground or in the air.

Over the last few decades, the circus has become a more appreciated form of entertainment. The most well-known of these is the private circus company named Cirque du Soleil. Formed in Montreal in 1984, Cirque du Soleil now performs on 5 continents and 200 cities and attracts 90 million spectators per year. The shows are well supported, with each show having 2–3 full-time physiotherapists to assist the performers.

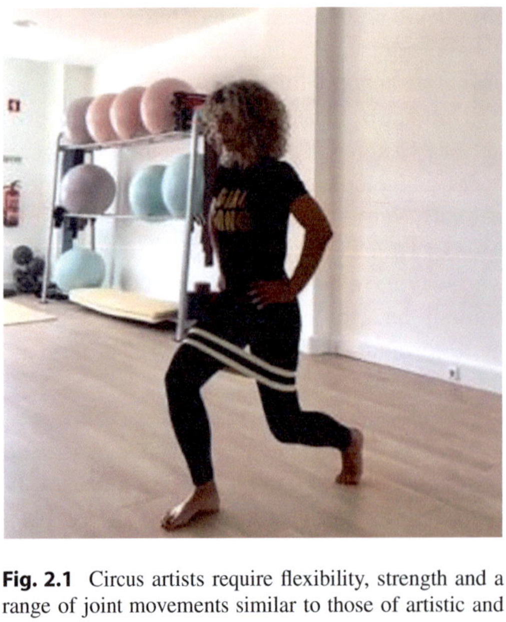

Fig. 2.1 Circus artists require flexibility, strength and a range of joint movements similar to those of artistic and rhythmic gymnastics

2.4 Epidemiology

Circus acts are different to gymnastic disciplines in many different aspects, which could influence injury patterns and also epidemiological studies. Within gymnastics, the emphasis is on competition with athletes training to perform at their best on one particular day, and much preparation is focused on that day. In the circus, emphasis is given to entertainment of the audience with complex, daring and apparently risky performances daily. Whereas gymnastic training may be modified in the presence of injury to peak on competition day, circus performers have to complete their routines day after day. Many will have little time to rest and recover from injuries before the next maximal effort is required.

Circuses traditionally tend to move from location to location to attract audiences in different cities. Only the most successful companies will have adequate resources of physiotherapy and rehabilitation, and these tend to be those who remain in one location and can draw large crowds night after night for an entire "season". Performers understand that with the finance at stake, "the show must go on" and that they may be encouraged or be required to perform with injuries. Similar to team sports, if replacements are found, it may be more difficult for an injured performer to get back into the cast or troupe.

Cirque du Soleil is probably considered to be the most professional circus company and has maintained databases of injury and illness data. Shrier et al. analysed presentations and treatments provided by the show's therapists over a 5-year period. One thousand three hundred and seventy-six artists sustained 18,336 show- or training-related injuries. Of the 6,70q injuries sustained, 80% required $\leq$7 treatments and resulted in $\leq$ missed performances. This presents an injury rate of 9.7 per 1000 athlete exposure. By contrast, the USA's National Collegiate Athletic Association's women's gymnastics team had had injury rate of 0.74 per 1000 athlete exposures.

Most of the injuries reported are minor, and the rates of more serious injuries are lower than those reported from NCAA participation. This study looked at only work-related complaints, and it needs to be noted that artists often have multiple roles within the show. Females tended to have a relatively larger number of hip and groin problems and so potentially may benefit from a prevention programme as part of their preparation. By contrast, musicians tended to report more distal injuries. Shrier and Hallé reported on a cohort study of 47 artists to determine psychological predictors of injuries in circus artists. Using a validated questionnaire, the authors reported that injury, emotional exhaustion, self-efficacy and fatigue are associated with increased injury risk.

As with all injury epidemiology reporting, terminology is a key component. Acute and chronic injury descriptions have been considered together with acrobat and non-acrobat, but in Hamilton's study, the terminology of sudden and non-sudden loading was used. The effect of injury was less on non-sudden load acts; however, medical attendance for treatment was similar.

Wanke et al. have analysed 17 years of data from the Berlin State Artist Educational School. Looking at 160 participants in the study, they found that injury risk was low with 0.3 injuries per 1000 hours of participation. Seven percent of injuries resulted in a break or absence of more than 3 days. Injury patterns depended upon the activity together with the use of props and equipment.

An injury study of participants at an Australian Circus School reported on 351 injuries requiring 1948 treatments in 63 students. They noted that females reported hip injuries more commonly, whereas in males, the most common sites injured were forearms and ankles. The time spent training in specific disciplines and contortions was also a factor.

Wolfenden and Angioi performed a systematic review to identify the musculoskeletal profile of circus artists, until March 2016. Eight studies were identified from the literature yielding a low injury rate of 7.4–9.3 per 1000 artist exposures. The spine and the back were the most frequently injured areas. Most injuries were soft tissue, requiring few treatments and few missed or altered performances with a low risk of re-injury.

Recent work by Stubbe et al. evaluated 44 circus arts students prospectively for 1 year, completing the Oslo Sports Trauma Research Centre questionnaire for health problems. There was an 82.9% response rate, with 70.5% of respondents reporting an injury and 19.5% illness and finally 5% mental health problems. The overall injury incidence rate was 3.3 per 1000 hours of participation. The most common site of injury was the shoulder 27.7%, and the average duration of absence due to injury was 6.9 days.

Finally, a qualitative study has looked at participants of Cirque du Soleil with a semi-structured interview. Injury was described as a performance limitation and related to physical load factors. In regard to injury prevention, this was localised to artist-related factors, e.g. technique and lifestyle together with the occurrence of physical load factors. The findings of this study were that shared responsibility and open communication among stakeholders were considered to be key factors for injury prevention (Fig. 2.2).

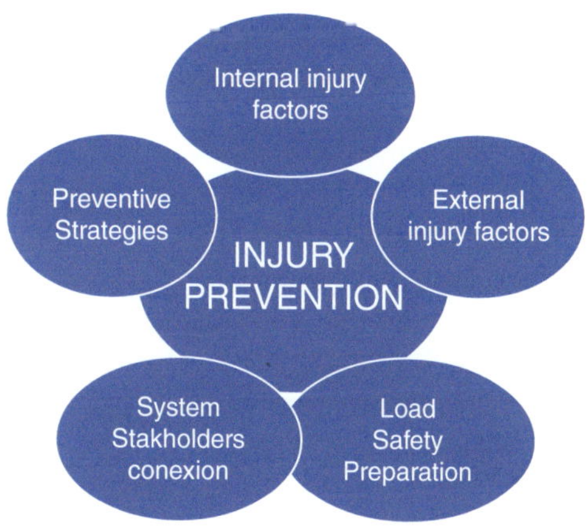

Fig. 2.2 A multilevel system map with factors strategies and stakeholders in relation to injuries and their prevention. (**a**) Artist-related intrinsic injury factors; (**b**) external injury factors; (**c**) main preventative strategies, e.g. load management, safety and preparation, which are driven by factors from the inner two circles; (**d**) stakeholders in the system as well as how they connect to the strategies and factors of multiple levels

2.5 Diagnosis

The diagnosis of injuries in the circus is no different to those in other sports and follows the common practice of resuscitation, history, physical examination, specific tests relating to the joint in question and imaging with plain radiographs and ultrasonography and magnetic resonance imaging. It is beyond the scope of this chapter to discuss these as individual specific injuries.

2.6 Medical Treatment of the Most Common Injuries

Treatment of the most common injuries require protect, optimal loading, ice, compression and elevation. Difficulties in the circus population, as already discussed, include the requirement for repeated aesthetic performances of a high-standard rather than an isolated optimal performance. This means that there may be limited opportunity to rest an injury or to have regular access to physiotherapy treatment. It is beyond the limit of this chapter to discuss the specifics of treatment, and there is no difference in treatment to that of artistic or rhythmic gymnastics.

2.7 Physiotherapy

For circus performers, a standard physiotherapy for sports injuries is recommended, with the difficulties and caveats already described. The author recommends consulting standard physiotherapy texts for this information, and it is beyond the scope of this chapter to discuss this further here.

2.8 Prevention

The circus is a prime performance activity for prevention programmes; however, many performers lack coaches with established qualifications, others acquired through years of experience within their art. From reviewing the literature above, prevention programmes for hip injuries for females and shoulder injuries for males are recommended.

Treatment may be hampered by frequent location moves and different therapists. One of the main problems with entertainment performance art is that if a performer is unable to complete their role, they may be replaced on a permanent basis.

2.9 Return to Performance

In common with many genres of performance art, it is the artist's perception of whether they are able to perform and additionally how aesthetic a performance looks. The risk of premature resumption of participation in performance must be balanced by the desire not to lose the artist's position and be replaced within the cast. Trapeze acts are akin to extreme sports when, given the risks involved, optimal performance is required, so for these performances, artists should only return once they are confident in their own ability to perform the act (Fig. 2.3).

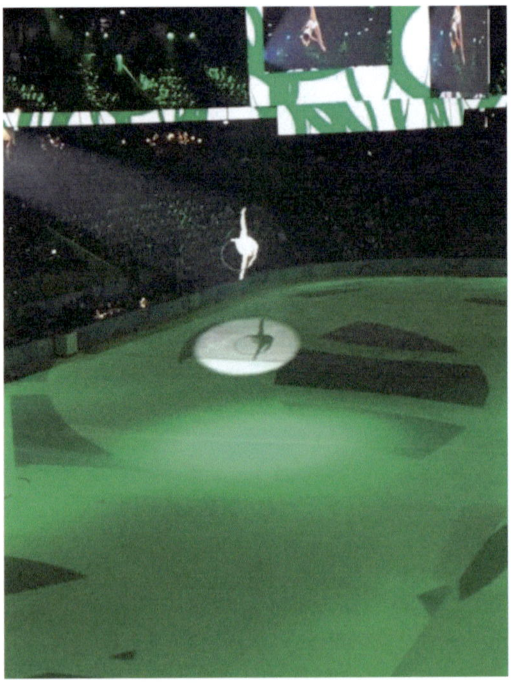

Fig. 2.3 A trapeze artist performing at the opening ceremony of the Winter Youth Olympic Games. At the dress rehearsal, an artist sustained critical injuries during a 5 m fall. This requires an immediate stunning, confidence in the presence of recent injury occurrence ability and aesthetics

2.10 Emergency Care

Whilst the provision on emergency care at gymnastic events is expected, there is no evidence to suggest this provision is made within circus acts. Professional extreme sports athletes ensure that safety is maintained; emergency extraction teams, e.g. helicopter, are available; and that hospitals are on standby. The athletes themselves ensure they are insured both medically and financially; however, there is little information in this regard relating to extreme performance art.

2.11 Summary

Contemporary circus is an acrobatic, athletic and aesthetic performance art which requires a high degree of training and presents an element of risk in the acute situation together with the risks of chronic injury with repetitive performance.

Bibliography

1. Shrier I, Meeuwisse WH, Matheson GO, et al. Injury patterns and injury rates in the circus acts: an analysis of 5 years of data from cirque du Soleil. Am J Sports Med. 2009;37(6):1143–9.
2. Hamilton GW, Meeuwisse WH, Emery CA, et al. Examining the effect of injury definition on risk factor analysis in circus artists. Scand J Med Sci Sport. 2012;22:330–4.
3. Wolfenden HEG, Angioi M. Musculoskeletal injury profile of circus artists: a systematic review of the literature. Med Probl Perform Art. 2017;32(1):51–9.
4. Bolling C, Melette J, Pasman HR, et al. From the safety net to the injury prevention web: applying systems thinking to unravel injury prevention challenges and opportunities in cirque du Soleil. BMJ Open Sport Exerc Med. 2019;5:e000492.

Upper Limb Disorders in Musicians

3

Paolo Arrigoni, Francesco Luceri,
Marco Passiatore, Emanuele Maggini,
and Giuseppe Milano

3.1 Introduction

Music plays an important role in human culture. Musicians, singers, and related workers hold approximately 249,000 jobs in the United States.

To achieve the necessary dexterity to become a high-level musician, it is necessary to put in many hours of training and improvement, which can take years of practice to reach "perfection."

Due to the high physical and psychological demands of their work, musicians have a high risk of developing a range of health problems. The main worry about health problems in musicians is that they can stop professional activity or that they can become potentially career-ending disabilities.

There are several specific groups of musicians depending on the musical instrument they play: string instrument, wind instrument, piano, and electronic keyboard or percussion instrument. Each of these groups has specific disorders, while some disorders occur equally in all groups. For example, musicians who play wind instruments can have dental stress and increased intraocular pressure, while those who play string instruments can have dermatitis and musculoskeletal disorders. Violinists and violists often suffer from pathological conditions in the jaw, back, neck, shoulder, and hands that can be either nerve related or muscular.

Playing a musical instrument involves a combination of repetitive and complicated movements that may cause musculoskeletal disorders over time. The neck, shoulder, and elbow are the most commonly affected areas. Repetitive work with a sustained abnormal posture and high forces are important in the development of upper-limb disorders in the workplace. It is necessary to warn musicians of the initial symptoms and how they can prevent the disorder from its worsening.

Zaza and Farewell [1] coined the definition "playing-related musculoskeletal disorders" (PMRDs) to highlight the occurrence of muscu-

P. Arrigoni
U.O. Clinica Ortopedica e Traumatologica Universitaria CTO, ASST Gaetano Pini-CTO, Milan, Italy

Laboratory of Applied Biomechanics, Department of Biomedical Sciences for Health, University of Milan, Milan, Italy

F. Luceri
Laboratory of Applied Biomechanics, Department of Biomedical Sciences for Health, University of Milan, Milan, Italy

M. Passiatore · G. Milano (✉)
Department of Medical and Surgical Specialties, Radiological Sciences, and Public Health, University of Brescia, Brescia, Italy

Department of Bone and Joint Surgery, Spedali Civili, Brescia, Italy

E. Maggini
Department of Bone and Joint Surgery, Spedali Civili, Brescia, Italy
e-mail: e.maggini001@unibs.it

H. Jones, A. Lukaszenko (eds.), *Injury Prevention and Care in Artistic Sports*,
https://doi.org/10.1007/978-3-032-18105-3_3

loskeletal disorders in musicians. The authors reported that a lot of professional and student instrumentalists suffered current "pain, weakness, numbness, tingling, or other symptoms that interfere with their ability to play their instrument at the level they are accustomed to" [1], which forms the definition of PRMDs.

The improved methods of diagnosis and treatment confirm that musical artists suffer from special problems related to their occupation and lifestyle and the establishment of health programs emphasizing an interdisciplinary approach to these issues are fundamental developments in musicians' occupational medicine. Unfortunately, professional musicians with upper limb pain and other performance-related musculoskeletal disorders have received little attention in the literature.

3.2 Epidemiology

Work-related musculoskeletal disorders are the most frequent complaints among instrumental musicians. They can cause pain, disability, and loss of employment. The prevalence of musculoskeletal disorders in instrumental musicians is high, ranging from 73.4% to 87.7%: the hands, shoulder, neck, jaw, and back are the most commonly affected body regions [2]. The impact of these complaints on the professional musician can be significant, seriously influencing physical, psychological, social, and financial aspects of daily life.

The musculoskeletal problems observed more often in musicians are overuse (50%), nerve compression or thoracic outlet syndrome (20%), and focal dystonia (10%).

The type of instrument seems to have unclear influence on the occurrence of physical discomfort, and epidemiological studies encountered very different results in terms of general prevalence of problems in a single instrument. String instrumentalists showed a prevalence of musculoskeletal problems in 69% of the cases, conditions of the peripheral nerves in 19%, focal dystonia in 5%, and others conditions in 7%. The viola and the double bass presented a higher proportion of individuals who had to interrupt the instrumental activity; sometimes, the violinists and violists are more affected by problems; sometimes, they present fewer symptoms [3].

3.3 Etiology

The musician is essentially a highly trained athlete, normally making specific use of hands and arms, although other parts of the body may be utilized in the playing of certain larger instruments. Most upper-limb injuries in musicians are caused by repetitiveness, inappropriate postures, and stress brought about by remaining seated for a long time or carrying instruments.

Pain is the main symptom of these lesions, and musicians who play string instruments are the most affected [4]. In the case of musicians, such as violinists, who have long and daily training routines, the repetitive movements they perform are forced, and sometimes, the postures are not natural [5].

Playing-related musculoskeletal complains very probably do not have one causal factor but are more likely a multifactorial issue. There are specific playing-related risk factors that should be explained. These can be divided into four categories: internal factors, external factors, physical factors, and instrumental factors [6].

3.3.1 Internal Factors

Internal factors may be considered those aspects of playing that are directly determined by the musician. A sudden increase in playing time is the most important risk factor. This is reflected by the fact that not so many musicians perform warming-up exercises [7]. Also, the intensity of practice is an important factor that contributes to musculoskeletal complains. Sudden changes in repertoire, technique, or instrument can simply exceed the physiological limits of an individual's musculoskeletal structure [6].

A physical warm-up and cooldown before and after playing is desirable and seen as being essential. The neck, shoulders, and arms should be the focus areas [8].

Age is another important element to analyze: musicians older than 30 years of age are more at risk.

3.3.2 External Factors

The most obvious external factor is stress and associated psychological dysfunction: performance anxiety, upcoming injuries, auditions, financial considerations, and the strict time of constraints of recording sessions are only some of the most common stress-inducing conditions in musicians [9].

3.3.3 Physical Factors

Women are more at risk than men for serious musculoskeletal problems [10]. This observation has been attributed to the smaller build and lower muscle power of females, as well as smaller hand size and a greater incidence of benign hypermobility that may represent an obvious manifestation of a genetic vulnerability of the soft tissues that puts an individual at risk. In addition, there is an evidence that tendons in women are stiffer than those in males. The combination of a loose joint with a stiff tendon may synergistically increase the risk for female musicians [6].

3.3.4 Instrumental Factors

The relationship between musicians and their instruments is the focal point of ergonomic analysis and biomechanical training [4]. It is known that the type of instrument is related to the occurrence of musculoskeletal complains among musicians. Usually violinist, violist, and pianists are mentioned as having the highest risk [10].

The aspects to take note that are important to evaluate the risk of an instrument are the posture maintained in playing, instrument weight, pressure of the instrument on contact points of the body of the performer, and the individual physiological demands, such as breath control.

Each instrument or class of instruments presents unique demands in all categories of risk factors [6]. For example, the work of violinists and violists requires a seated position throughout the entire rehearsal and performance period. They look for the best body position, seeking balance and distribution of body weight to obtain greater motor control and precision of movements in the instrumental execution. The violin and the viola require an extreme external shoulder rotation position, arm elevation and constant maximum supination of the left forearm, which can lead to bursitis and tendinopathics of the shoulder muscles. The consequent load on the tendons of the muscles adjacent to the shoulder can cause overuse injuries, and it should be considered that continuous arm elevation increases intramuscular pressure. Flexors and extensors of the right hand are used to control the bow and the muscles that keep the left hand in ulnar deviation, and the finger extensors can also present overuse. Symptomatic violinists and violists can alter their technique to reduce the force caused by the instrument on the jaw, reducing pain and dysfunction.

3.4 Shoulder Disorders in Musicians

The diagnosis of specific shoulder diseases affecting musicians is often very difficult. Acute lesions directly caused by making music are rare. The most frequent injuries of musicians are caused by an imbalance between load and load-bearing capacity, excessive use (overuse), or incorrectly (misuse), making music. Mostly are chronic conditions with a long-lasting history, making the diagnosis often very difficult.

The initial symptoms that often appear are pain, in about 85% of cases, heavy limb, burning sensation, and tiredness in one or more parts of the body and may arise even after a short period of activity [11]. Furthermore, the neurological examination is characteristically normal, with no sensory or reflex abnormalities [12].

Musicians' injuries are often caused by a sudden change in the "musical load" or intensity of playing. Possible sources may be a change in the teacher, instruments, repertoire, or practical habits. Beware of a sudden change after a holiday or in preparation for a concert, audition or examination, or speed exercises with the metronome. Any change in the "musical load" is a risk factor and is important to recognize for diagnosis purposes.

Clinical evaluation is based on classical principles with the evaluation of posture, the presence of dyskinesias, the range of motion (ROM), rotator cuff function, and trigger point sensitivity. Postural evaluation during specific musical activity of the patient may be useful. Physical exam must also include the classic tests for rotator headsets (Whipple, Jobe, Apley, etc.) and specific tests as Neer impingement test and Hawking-Kennedy test for subacromial impingement, Kibler's lateral slide test for scapular dyskinesias, and Beighton's test for hypermobility (Fig. 3.1).

Musicians' diseases can be divided into organic and non-organic problems. In organic problems, there can be tenosynovitis, shoulder impingement, hypermobility syndrome (HMS), and osteoarthritis. On the other side, non-organic problems such as overuse syndrome, thoracic outlet syndrome, and focal dystonia are more work related [13]. Lockwood described that overuse syndrome is the most common cause of upper-extremity symptoms related to playing [14].

Although much attention has been paid on peripheral mechanisms of pain, newer theories are considering occupational pain as the manifestation of motor control conflicts between postural static supporting muscle activity and rhythmic, skilled, repetitious, dynamic muscle activity [15].

3.4.1 Rotator Cuff Injury

Musicians that repetitively use their hands overhead, such as small string instrument players (e.g., violin), are susceptible to rotator cuff injury. Usually, when tendons are stressed beyond their limits, microscopic tearing occurs, which stimulate an inflammatory response to induce tendon healing. However, when the tendons are not given time to heal before they are subjected to the same activity, as it happens in music players, the inflammation becomes chronic, and proper healing does not occur, establishing a rotator cuff tendinosis. This type of inflammation not only can cause pain but can also lead to progressive damage of the tendons themselves.

In the literature, we can describe two theories than can explain the development of rotator cuff injuries. The classical theory by Neer (1972) tells that there is a mechanical rubbing of the rotator cuff against the acromion during arm elevation over the head, which can lead to the inflammation and tears of the tendons. On the other hand, there

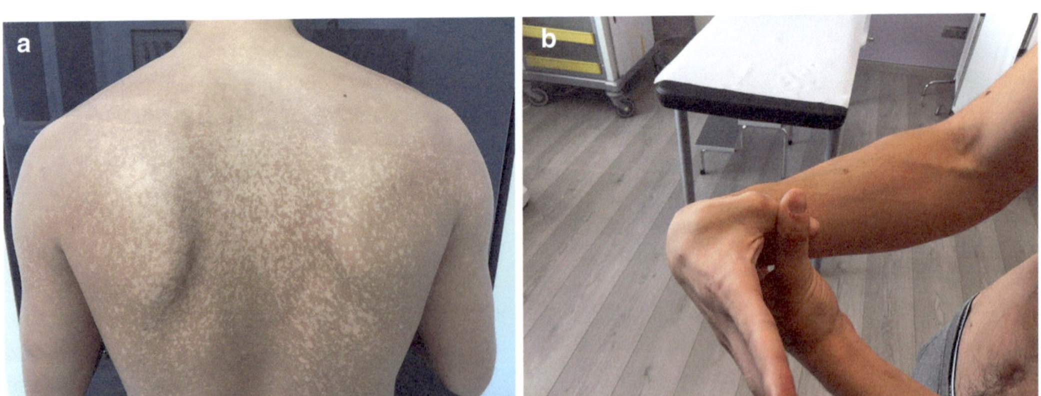

Fig. 3.1 (**a**) Scapula dyskinesis (left) with prominence of the medial border. (**b**) Joint hypermobility must be tested

is a second theory by Uhthoff (1997) describing that there is a primary degeneration of the rotator cuff tendon itself [16].

The muscle mostly involved in rotator cuff complex is supraspinatus. In the right shoulder of the violin and flute players, this muscle is wounded by the prolonged positions of abduction or static flexion of the forearm; in the left shoulder, the muscle belly is injured by the flexion and adduction of the shoulder itself. Infraspinatus and teres minor are less implicated in this process: they are involved when the right shoulder is in maximal abduction of 80° [5].

The main symptom of rotator cuff tendonitis is pain, which tends to worsen when the patient lifts the arm over the shoulder or during the night. Repetitive or sustained arm activity over time can cause distress to the patient as well as weakness in certain arm positions such as external rotation and forward flexion [16].

3.4.2 Overuse Syndrome

In literature, there are many different definitions of overuse syndrome (OS). For some authors, overuse injury, repetitive strain injury, cumulative trauma disorder, and repetitive motion injury may be considered all synonyms for the effects on the soft tissues of "repeated or continuous application of slight to moderate physical stress over extended periods of time" [17].

Lederman and Calabrese [18] consider involvement of any soft tissue including tendon, tendon sheath, ligament, muscle, nerve, or synovium bursa. Fry [19] limits his definition in describing an "overuse syndrome" as the painful musculoligamentous injury caused by physical activity. He excludes other specific entities such as tenosynovitis and nerve entrapments. Other authors define the OS like a clinical entity in its own right, caused by overload or repetition of some movements giving episodes of microtrauma to muscle and joint ligaments, resulting in chronic inflammation and fibrosis as connective tissue is slowly taken beyond its biomechanical and physiological limits [20–22].

As a result, presenting in various ways, e.g., neuropathy, tendonitis, tenosynovitis, peritendinitis, crepitans, arthritis, spondylosis, reflex sympathetic dystrophy, or repetitive stress lesions (RSI), one can deduce how difficult the diagnosis is to make.

Pain represents the most important symptom of OS in musicians, but it can be anticipated by prodromes like stiffness, discomfort, tingling, functional loss and, occasionally, paresthesia in the affected part. Tenderness may be elicited over the contractile structures without other signs of franc inflammation. But later, these problems, without an appropriate treatment, will progress, giving a reduction in shoulder strength, muscle wasting, and, possibly, tenosynovitis.

Fry [23] developed a useful functionally oriented grading system for overuse syndrome that includes signs and symptoms divided in five grades:

- Grade 1. Pain in one site only while playing.
- Grade 2. Pain in multiple sites.
- Grade 3. Pain that persists well beyond the time that the musician stops playing.
- Grade 4. All of the above plus activities of daily living (ADL) beginning to cause pain.
- Grade 5. All of the above plus all daily activities that engage the affected body part causing pain.

The causes of this syndrome seem to be associated with a change in technique or increase in playing time. There are two different mechanisms for OS that have been theorized and can explain why string players are more at risk. The first considers injury to muscle under static low-level loads. This is common in shoulders as they work as essential fixators, holding instrument in the correct position. For the majority of string instrumentalists, the weight of the instrument is supported in whole or part by their shoulders, whereas wind players need to support the weight of their instrument with their fingers or thumbs only. The second proposed mechanism is injury to other structures, such as tendon sheaths, under high repetition activities. This occurs directly in the fingers and the muscles that move them. Playing stringed instruments requires strength and force to hold down the string, followed by rapid release to move to the next note position. This may involve a change in wrist position as well as movement up and down the neck of the instrument. Comparatively, less force is required to hold the key of a wind instrument, and generally, only the fingers need to move as the hand is statically maintained in the correct position [24].

3.4.3 Shoulder Impingement

It is a common type of overuse syndrome, in which the rotator cuff tendons and the subacromial bursa are entrapped in the subacromial space, between the bony acromial arch and the humeral head. Compression of the biceps tendon may also be involved.

Activity that require positions of shoulder in abduction and flexion and use of these larger muscles (such as cello playing) place the rotator cuff's muscles and scapular stabilizers under increased load in order to maintain stability of the shoulder joint. If control and strength of muscles is not enough, this can lead to the upward movement of the humeral head, causing painful impingement of the supraspinatus tendon and the subacromial bursa between the acromion and the head of the humerus. If the activity causing impingement is not modified or the underlying muscular imbalances are not addressed, shoulder impingement can lead to a rotator cuff tear whereby the supraspinatus tendon becomes frayed through abrasion against the acromion (Fig. 3.2).

Known risk factors for impingement include work tasks that involve repetitive motion and positions that take large amounts of shoulder abduction and flexion [25]. All these requirements are consistent with string players bowing movements, and motion capture studies on string bow arms suggest that this increased load may lead to the high levels of shoulder dysfunction seen in this population [26].

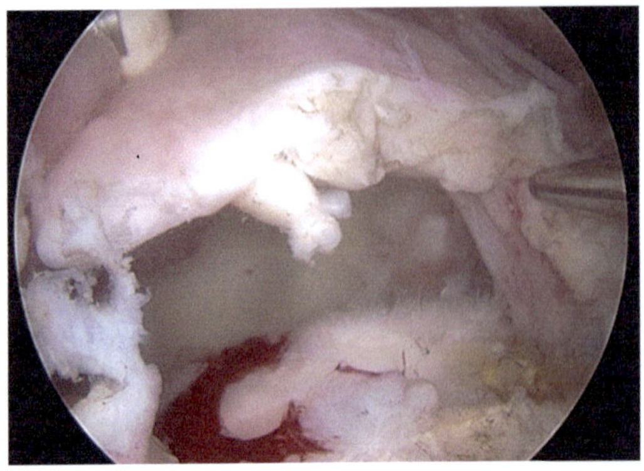

Fig. 3.2 Shoulder impingement can lead to a rotator cuff tear whereby the supraspinatus tendon becomes frayed through abrasion against the acromion

Age is also a common predictor of impingement; the most common age range for this type of lesion is 18–40 years. Impingement does not discriminate between the sexes, affecting men and women equally (unlike other shoulder diseases) [27].

The most significant subjective feature of shoulder impingement is the report of pain, or a painful arc of movement, particularly with overhead arm movement. The painful arc usually occurs between 60° and 120° of shoulder abduction. Some authors have also reported night pain as a clinical feature. Other physical signs include palpation tenderness over the greater tuberosity, supraspinatus tendon, and the anterior edge of the acromion. Neer impingement test is highly reliable in establishing a clinical diagnosis of shoulder impingement.

Surprisingly, in violin players, it was noted that shoulder pain is present less frequently in the bowing arm (right) than in the instrument-supporting arm (left).

It is also interesting to note that the music students may be more predisposed to develop shoulder impingement than professionals. Fry suggested that students tend to use larger muscle groups when playing, such as the deltoid and pectoralis, while professionals are more relaxed and use the smaller rotator muscle groups [28].

3.4.4 Thoracic Outlet Syndrome

Thoracic outlet syndrome is a condition characterized by the compression of the arteries, nerves, or veins in the zone between the lower neck and the axilla.

Up to 45% of all nerve entrapments in musicians are identified as this syndrome. We can describe four common anatomical regions of potential involvement: the cervical rib, the anterior scalene muscle, the clavicle and the first rib, the pectoralis minor muscle, and the first rib.

The usual neurological manifestation involves the lower trunk (C8–T1), with the forearm and hand pain and paresthesia in the ulnar territory.

Lederman [29] described the maneuver to identify the specific anatomic localization of the disease; the arm must be downward tractioned and internally rotated. Fifty percent were noted to have droopy shoulders, and many authors found that instrument playing aggravated these neurological symptoms.

Vascular syndromes, while much less common, have been reported in musicians: subclavian artery stenosis in cellists and axilla-subclavian vein obstruction in violinists [6].

3.4.5 Hypermobility Syndrome

Hypermobility syndrome (HMS) is a comorbidity related to the enlarged range of motion of joints [13]. It has a higher prevalence in musicians compared to the general population: it may have beneficial and disadvantageous effects for music playing. This condition can increase the risk of musculoskeletal damage during specific exercises.

Larsson et al. [30] found that violinist and flautist with hypermobility feel less musculoskeletal problems in wrist and hand region compared to musicians without this condition. However, related to joints where stability is required, such as the shoulder, hypermobility could induce inadequate control due to excessive ROM and increased muscle tension needed to stabilize the instrument.

To prevent shoulder injuries, the core of the therapeutic regimen is based on strengthening exercises and warm-up [9].

3.4.6 Conservative Treatment

The most important role in these patients is certainly played by conservative treatment. Early specialized medical assessment (with the musical instrument) is essential and must be an integral part of the conservative treatment plan.

Conservative therapy should be based on a holistic approach to patient health. The musician must be aware of the pathologies she/he may face and must know how to prevent and treat these conditions.

Therapeutic conversation with extensive explanation and advice can be very useful. It is also very important for the physician to sensitize the patient to healthy lifestyle, improvement of blood circulation and core stability by general physical fitness training, and, if applicable, completely stop smoking.

Relative rest with frequent short breaks and sufficient recovery time is the principal treatment in overuse injuries. Evidence as far back as the nineteenth century suggests the most useful treatment for OS is rest. However, rest means different things to different people, and the physician should explain how they expect the patient to interpret this. It may be a decrease in playing time, a change in technique, or complete cessation of playing and, if possible, practicing other activities regarded as contributory [22]. However, the muscle atrophy and bone wasting that occurs with enforced rest may create additional problems [31]. Therefore, gymnastics must be taken into account.

Physical and postural therapies play an important role, and musicians should pay attention to playing posture, stabilization of the trunk and shoulder belt, and practical habits. Endurance training, with free weights, elastics or tubing, or exercise machines, prepares the musician for long hours of training and performance and helps ensure that muscles and joints are more than equal to the stresses and strains required. Exercises should be performed very gently and within a painless range. The postures should be inserted slowly and maintained for 30–60 s.

By specifically entering into shoulder pathology, knowledge of shoulder blade position during shoulder mobility exercises can help the patient establish better models of shoulder stability. The patient may need to be trained to involve the latissimus dorsi, elevator scapulae, rhomboids, and rotator cuff muscles in sequence (Fig. 3.3).

Among the progressive resistive exercises, ROM exercises of the shoulder against gravity is the main one. Codman exercises are a widely used program to improve the range of shoulder movement. When the individual is painless, low free-weight exercises are added and advanced slowly. Isometric exercises on the shoulders, elbows, and wrists are added with attention to the musician's ability to limit fatigue or pain by limiting effort.

Adaptation of the musical instrument and ergonomic sitting when playing should become a common practice. For example, simple and useful aids can be used such as changing shoulder support or chin rest on the violin, lengthening the c-c-c-sharp key and g-g-sharp key on a flute or bent flute, or a thumb rest adapted for oboe or clarinet. In addition, a suitable, ergonomic, and adjustable seat for the musician and the specific instrument used can allow the feet to be firmly planted on the floor with the ankles, knees, and hips at an angle of 90 degrees, supporting lumbar lordosis.

Other forms of conservative therapy can be cryotherapy, cortisone injections and non-steroidal anti-inflammatory drugs (NSAIDs), and immobilization or stabilization with tape, braces, or splints.

3.4.7 Surgical Treatment

Surgical treatment is rarely necessary for shoulder diseases in musicians and, if necessary, does not deviate from the common therapy for the general population. Surgical therapy tends to be achieved only when conservative therapy fails and there is an objective evidence of anatomic lesions. Nevertheless, it is quite common that professional musicians may not be able to afford the convalescent downtime following surgery; some may desire intervention early to allow a fast return to high-level playing. The role of arthroscopy in the diagnosis and surgical treatment of shoulder disorders is evolving. Arthroscopic subacromial decompression in the treatment of chronic stage II impingement syndromes is debated, while early repair of partial or full-thickness rotator cuff repair is strongly indicated to achieve satisfactory subjective and functional results and to prevent worsening of rotator cuff tear over time. Patients with massive and irreparable cuff tears have achieved significant pain relief from arthroscopic decompression and debridement of the floppy and irregular cuff margins.

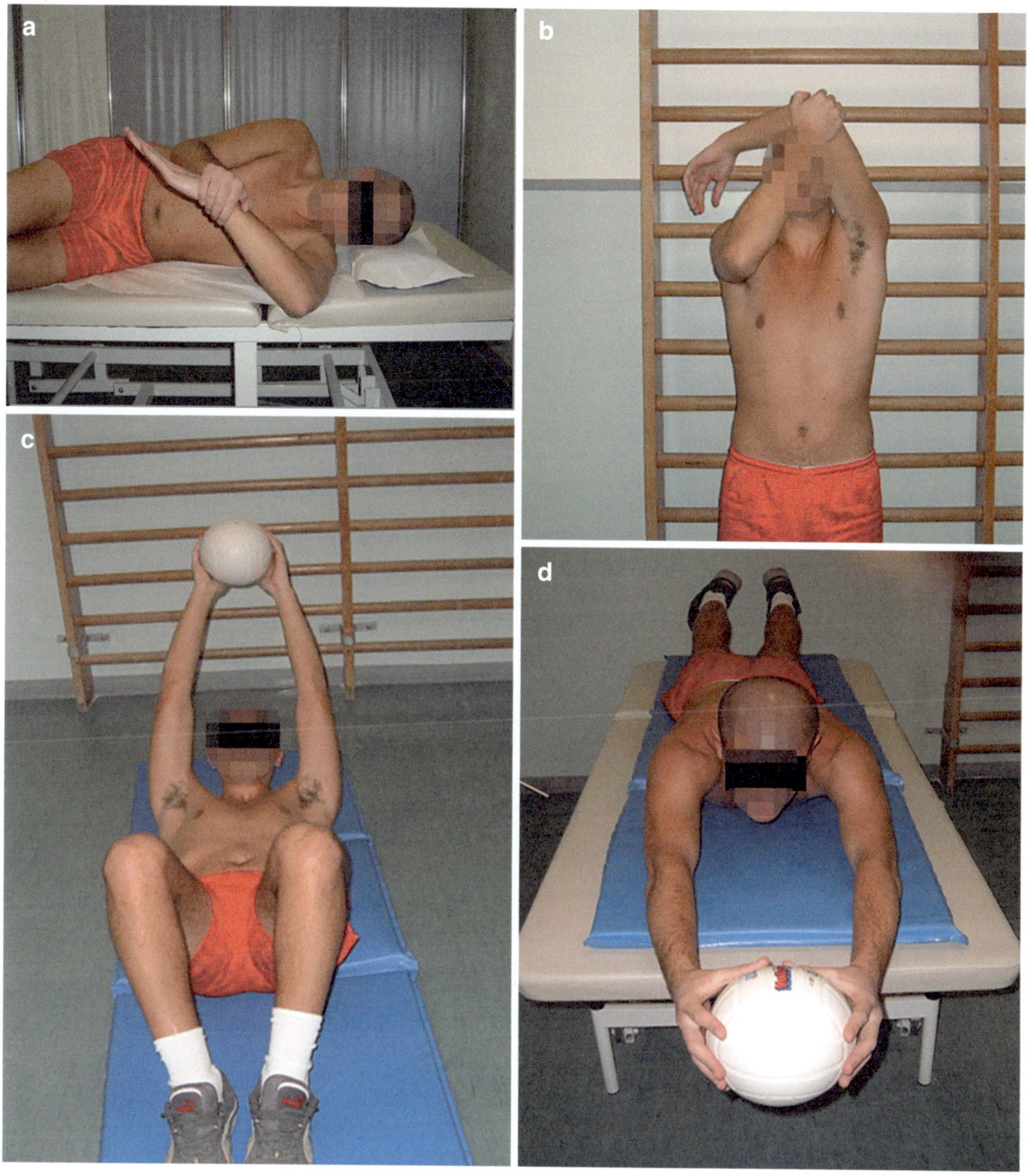

Fig. 3.3 Core rehabilitation is crucial to improve strength and neuromuscular control of scapular stabilizers. Standard program consists of capsular stretching (**a**, **b**); strengthening of abdominal (**c**) and lumbopelvic (**d**) muscles; closed-kinetic chain (**e**, **f**) and open-kinetic chain (**g**, **h**) isometric exercises for scapular stabilizers; deltoid and rotator cuff strengthening exercises (**i**, **j**); proprioceptive exercises to restore equilibrium (**k**); plyometric exercises for power and speed (**l**); and kinesthetic exercises for neuromuscular control (**m**)

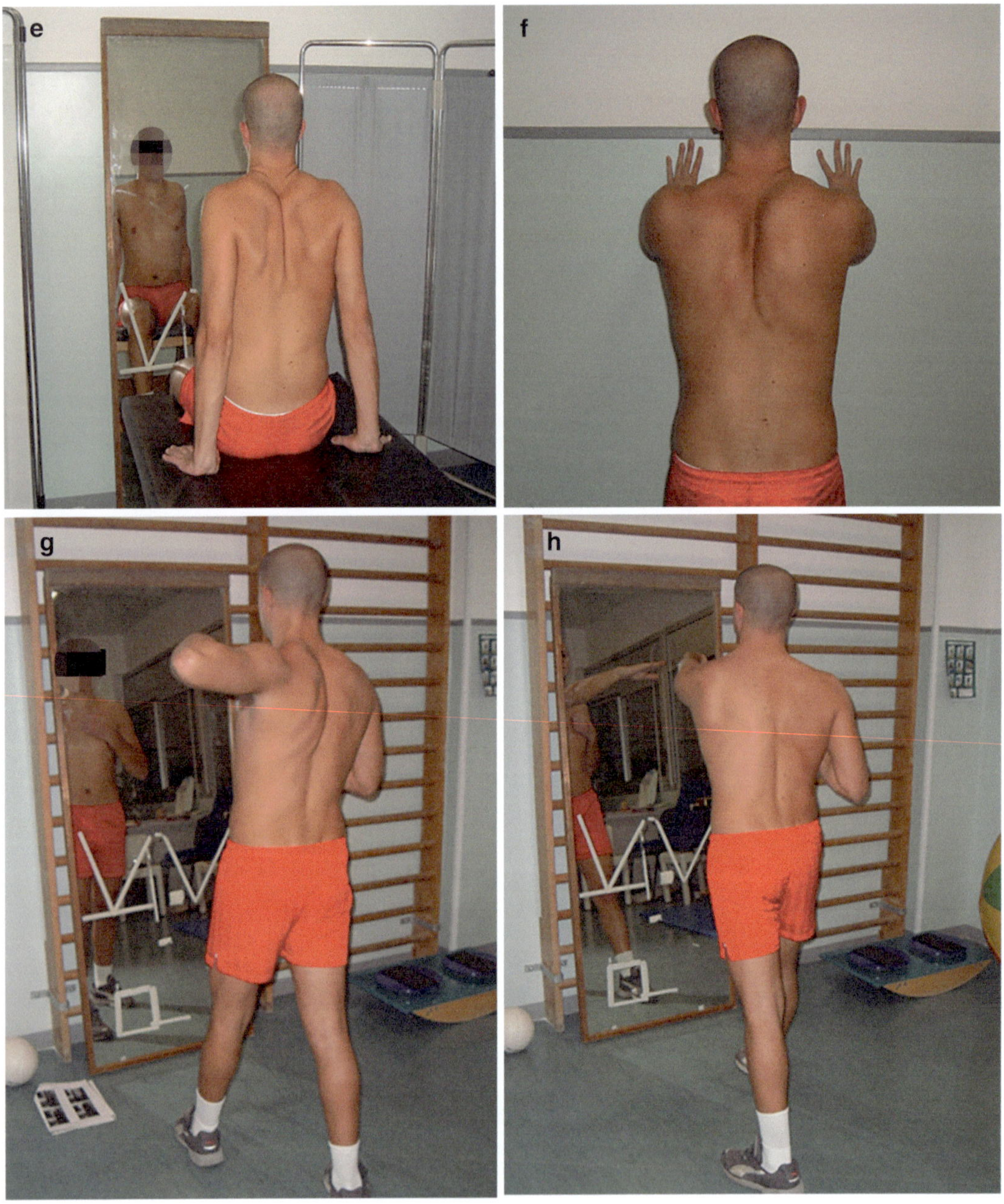

Fig. 3.3 (continued)

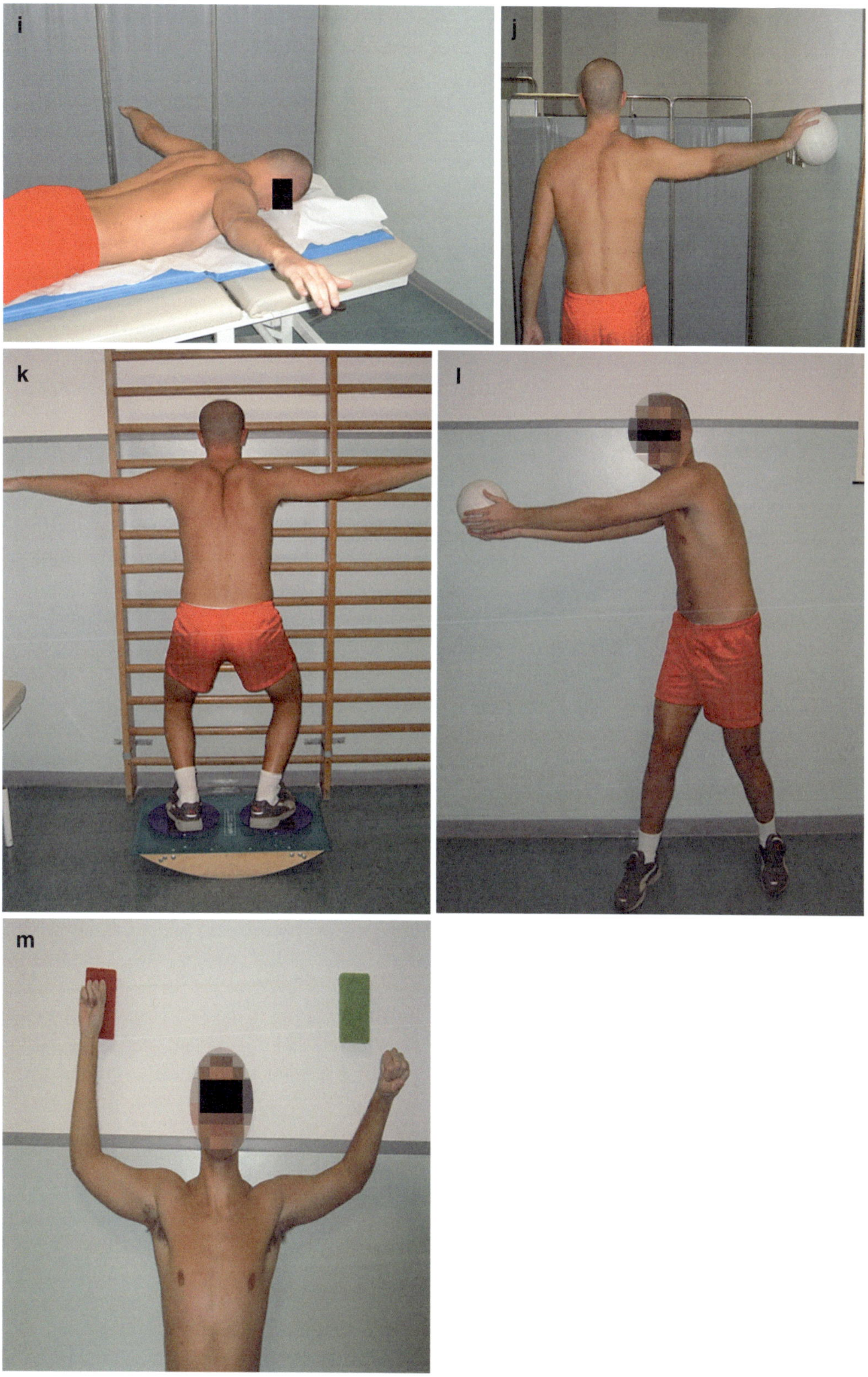

Fig. 3.3 (continued)

3.5 Elbow and Wrist Disorders in Musicians

There are several common conditions in the elbow and wrist that are caused or exacerbated by work-related exposures in musicians. Three diagnoses predominate in the medical literature: overuse syndrome, entrapment neuropathy, and functional dystonia. Disorders that should be considered include lateral and medial epicondylitis, wrist tenosynovitis, carpal tunnel syndrome, and de Quervain's tenosynovitis, all of which can cause forearm pain and can be work related.

3.5.1 Diagnosis

The musician's consultation comprises a similar work-up as any patient starting with history, physical examination, and possibly additional studies. For the physician to have some knowledge of playing a music instrument is desirable. If possible, let the musician take their instrument to the office visit. This allows observation of their playing technique, instrument hold, and posture.

Pain is the most frequent symptom leading musicians to consult a physician. In approximately one third of playing-related musculoskeletal disorders (PMRD), a specific diagnosis as carpal tunnel syndrome or epicondylitis can be defined. However, in the larger part, no specific diagnosis can be made, and the symptoms better fit a broader definition as regional pain syndrome or "non-specific forearm pain" (NSFP) [1, 32, 33].

Regional pain syndrome, as defined by Lederman [12], defines a combination of symptoms that comprises pain or tenderness at one or more locations in the forearm, primarily in the muscles rather than the joints or tendons, accompanied by tightness, stiffness, cramping, fatigue, swelling, or paresthesia. Pain can be elicited by stretching or activating the affected muscle-tendon unit against resistance. A similar diagnosis first mentioned by MacIver et al. [33] is NSFP, which refers to diffuse pain in the forearm in absence of diagnostic physical signs. There may be non-specific tenderness and possible loss of dexterous movements. In order to diagnose NSFP, it is essential to firstly exclude other conditions that could mimic this condition (i.e., epicondylitis, carpal tunnel syndrome, de Quervain's tenosynovitis).

Focal dystonia, or musician's cramp, is a rare but very invalidating neurological condition that causes the muscle in a specific part of the body to involuntarily contract or hold abnormal postures. For example, the musician's fingers can involuntarily hold a flexed position or oppositely an extended position that limits them from appropriately playing their instrument. It has an insidious onset and causes difficulty with control, speed, or dexterity for the musician [34].

Table 3.1 describes an overview of the common diagnoses in musicians presenting with wrist or elbow problems, including their cause, accompanying symptoms, and specific physicals tests. Although less likely do exclude specific diagnoses prior to diagnosing NFSP by physical examination, specific tests, and possibly adding electromyography or nerve conduction studies in the work-up for nerve entrapment syndromes. Be aware that the latter may be falsely negative, especially if symptoms are variably present or mild.

Physical examination is like that of regular patients and comprises visual inspection and palpation of the entire upper extremity, including the cervical spine. Search for limb asymmetry, muscular atrophy, and abnormal posture. Often it is important to observe the patient while performing to pinpoint the problem, so ask the musician to bring their instrument with them to the office if possible. For the trained eye, what can be recognized from playing is an inefficient posture, excessive tension, and extraneous movements.

3.5.2 Prevention

Education is important both for the patient, the attending physician, and the employer. The factors that predispose to illness are sudden increase of sessions playing the instrument, inadequate exercise regimen, incorrect playing habits such as lack of warm-up and stretching of muscles, the

Table 3.1 Overview of possible diagnoses in musicians presenting with wrist or elbow complaints

Condition	Cause	Symptoms	Specific test
Regional pain syndrome/ non-specific forearm pain (NSFP)	Overuse/postural/instrument	Diffuse forearm pain	–
Focal dystonia (musician's cramp)	Overuse/unclear	Difficulty with control, speed, or dexterity along with possible stiffness, cramping, tightness, and/or fatigue of the affected body part; occasional pain	–
Specific			
Medial epicondylitis	(Micro)tears common flexor origin at the medial epicondyle	Local tenderness at or just distal to the medial epicondyle and pain on resisted flexion of the wrist	
Lateral epicondylitis	(Micro)tears common extensor origin at the lateral epicondyle	Local tenderness at or just distal to the lateral epicondyle and pain on resisted extension of the wrist or gripping activities	
de Quervain's tenosynovitis	Tenosynovial inflammation of the first dorsal compartment, including the abductor pollicis longus and extensor pollicis brevis	Radial sided wrist pain. Pain with resisted thumb extension	Finkelstein's maneuver
Wrist tenosynovitis	Inflammation of the extensor or flexor sheaths at the wrist	Pain associated with movement of the affected tendon sheath in the wrist	
Nerve entrapment			
Carpal tunnel syndrome	Compression of the median nerve at the carpal tunnel	Pain, paresthesia, or sensory loss in the median nerve distribution; nocturnal exacerbation. Motor loss with atrophy of abductor pollicis brevis muscle if chronic	Tinel's test Phalen's maneuver Durkan's test (median nerve compression test)
Ulnar nerve entrapment at the elbow (i.e., cubital tunnel syndrome)	Compression of the ulnar nerve around the elbow	Pain, paresthesia, or sensory loss in the ulnar distribution (elbow, ulnar-sided forearm till hand); weakness and atrophy of ulnar-innervated muscles if chronic	Tinel's test Froment's sign Elbow flexion test
Thoracic outlet syndrome (neurogenic)	Compression of the brachial plexus	Pain, sensory symptoms (paresthesia, numbness), feeling of strength loss and/or fatigue on the affected side; any location in the interval from neck to arm; often position related (hyperabduction, abduction and extension)	Adson's test Wright's test

technical issues of the instrument such as grip with excessive force or tension, change of instrument, inadequate rehabilitation of previous injuries, postures, and inappropriate use of the body. Issues of individual and gender-related anatomical variability, use of improper chairs, execution of extra-musical activities that produce muscle tension, quality of the instruments used, and conditions of the room, with low lighting and temperature, are also important factors. Changes of repertoire or of instrument are also risk factors. The repertoire is considered a critical parameter in relation to the levels of force and pressure produced during the performance, interacting with the accessories added to the instrument, such as the chin rest.

Reduction of practice time, warm-up prior to playing, incorporation of rest periods during training sessions, correction of improper techniques, adequate eating habits, and hydration aid in the prevention of injuries. The provision of adequate information to musicians, ergonomic attitudes represented by adequate posture at home and at work, and use of appropriate furniture and awareness regarding postural problems as a means of disease prevention are also useful.

It is possible to prevent work-related disorders in musicians by analyzing the principal factors responsible for their development, such as poor posture, intensive practice, change in technique, inappropriate lifestyle, and anxiety. Musicians should be familiar with the anatomic and physiologic principles, which create their disabilities, and should also be educated about techniques of body movement, posture, and breathing. They should exercise regularly. They should also learn about the basic anatomy of playing an instrument as well as developing ways to manage stress and anxiety.

Table 3.2 Risk factors for developing PRMD [1, 4, 5]

Patient characteristics	Age
	Female
	Joint laxity
Biomechanical/ postural	Sudden increase in practice sessions/duration
	Inadequate exercise regimen
	Inappropriate posture/poor playing posture
	Inappropriate instrument hold
	Inappropriate use of body
Instrumental	Instrument type
	Instrument quality
	Change of instrument
	Change of repertoire
	No or improper use of instrument accessories (i.e., chin rest)
Preventative	Lack of warm-up
	Lack of cooldowns
	Lack of muscle stretching
	Lack of physical conditioning
	Inadequate rehabilitation of previous injury
Playing circumstances	Temperature (cold)
	Lighting (low)
	Improper chair
Psychosocial	Performance anxiety
	Depression
	Personal traits
	Work-related stress

3.5.3 Conservative Treatment

The etiology of PRMD is multifactorial and can be associated with poor posture, non-ergonomic instrument techniques, use of excessive force, and insufficient rest. In addition, the aspects of instrument shape and size, the duration of rehearsals, and workplace environment can contribute to the development of PRMD. An overview of risk factors for developing PRMDs is reported in Table 3.2 [1]. Symptoms usually begin to appear when the musician increases the intensity and duration of instrument use and rehearsal periods.

The majority of PRMDs, including above-mentioned specific diagnoses and nerve entrapment disorders, can be treated conservatively. Nerve entrapment syndromes have the highest treatment success rate, followed by regional pain syndromes. Unfortunately, treatment of focal dystonia remains largely unsuccessful [34].

Due to lack of widely accepted definitions and lack of standardized scientific research regarding PRMDs, there are no evidence-based guidelines for the treatment of the disorders [32]. Nonoperative treatment comprises of standard modalities as activity modification/rest, NSAIDs/analgesia, splinting, physical/occupational therapy, steroid injections, workplace modification, and addressing psychological features. Do not hesitate to involve the music teacher in the treatment process, as their knowledge on playing technique, instrument hold, and posture often exceeds that of the physician and may help in identifying technical or postural flaws. The latter can then be addressed during physical or occupational therapy.

Modifications of incorrect technique, changes in playing habits, periods of rest, training of correct postures, frequent stretching exercises, and adequate use of instrument accessories (i.e., chin or shoulder rests) are helpful in the treatment of PRMD.

The first aim of conservative treatment is to get rid of the pain using rest and activity modification perhaps in combination with analgesia. In case of nerve entrapment disorders, NSAIDs or (nightly) splinting may aid in reaching this goal.

Second, treatment should focus on conditioning and building resistance with physical or occupational therapy. Implementing periods of rest and stretching exercises, altering faulty playing habits, modifications of incorrect technique, and postural training all aid in the prevention of PRMDs. Also address use of instrument accessories (i.e., chin rest, shoulder rest) for biomechanical advantages, and optimize the work environment (temperature, lighting, chairs) to reduce work-related stress. Last, do not underestimate the psychological stresses that musicians are exposed to, especially in periods prior to performances, auditions, or examinations, and the possible disastrous consequences a PRMD may have for (aspiring) professional musicians (loss of income, cancellation of performances). The involvement of a psychologist may help reduce these stresses and unwanted muscle tension, aiding in the prevention of recurrences.

Nerve entrapment syndromes have the highest treatment success rate, followed by regional pain syndromes. Unfortunately, focal dystonia remains largely treated unsuccessfully.

3.5.4 Surgical Treatment

There is little evidence for the effectiveness of specific interventions to treat these pathologies. In cases in which physiotherapy, splints, topical medicines, and steroid injections are all administered without good results, it may be considered the surgical option.

Arthroscopy is recommended in the treatment of most of the elbow pathologies, such as arthroscopic release of the extensor carpi radialis brevis tendon for lateral epicondylitis and capsular repair accomplished with absorbable sutures in cases of posterolateral rotatory instability. Removal of loose bodies associated with joint locking and clicking, arthroscopic synovectomy, debridement, capsular excision, osteophyte removal, olecranon fossa fenestration, and possible radial head excision have been used in the arthroscopic treatment of osteoarthritis (Fig. 3.4). This procedure has been shown to have similar functional outcomes as an open approach, with patients returning to work sooner and having less postoperative therapy needs.

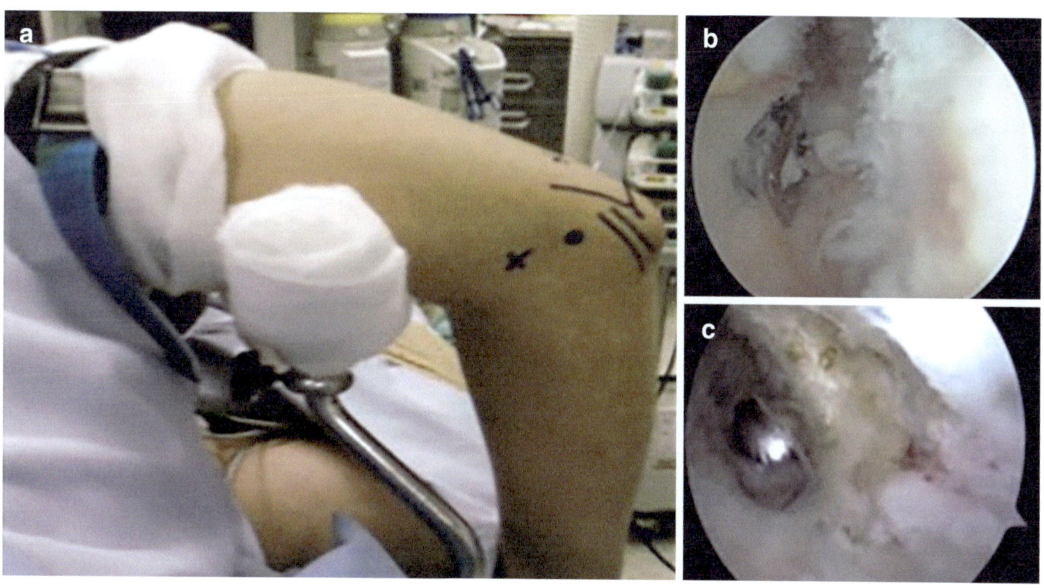

Fig. 3.4 (**a**) Elbow arthroscopy setting, (**b**) Stiff elbow: anterior capsulectomy. (**c**) Hypertrophic degenerative elbow: osteophyte removal

References

1. Zaza C, Farewell VT. Musicians' playing-related musculoskeletal disorders: an examination of risk factors. Am J Ind Med. 1997;32(3):292–300.
2. Rensing N, Schemmann H, Zalpour C. Musculoskeletal demands in violin and Viola playing: a literature review. Med Probl Perform Art. 2018;33(4):265–74.
3. Frank A, von Mühlen CA. Queixas musculoesqueléticas em músicos: Prevalência e fatores de risco. Rev Bras Reumatol. 2007;47(3):188–96.
4. Moraes GFS, Antunes AP. Musculoskeletal disorders in professional violinists and violists. Systematic review. Acta Ortopedica Brasileira. 2012;20(1):43–7.
5. Islan M, et al. Analysis and fem simulation methodology of dynamic behavior of human rotator cuff in repetitive routines: musician case study. J Med Syst. 2018;42(3):55.
6. Brown SE. Shoulder pain and the instrumental musician. J Back Musculoskelet Rehabil. 1992;2(2):16–27.
7. Kok LM, Haitjema S, Groenewegen KA, et al. The influence of a sudden increase in playing time on playing-related musculoskeletal complaints in high-level amateur musicians in a longitudinal cohort study. PLoS One. 2016;11(9)
8. Butler K, Norris R. Assessment and treatment principles for the upper extremities of instrumental musicians. In: Rehabilitation of the hand and upper extremity. Elsevier Health Sciences; 2011. p. 1859–61.
9. Sataloff RT, Brandfonbrener AG, Lederman RJ. Textbook of performing arts medicine. New York: Raven Press; 1991. p. 25–69.
10. Kok LM, Huisstede BMA, Nelissen RGHH. Musculoskeletal complaints in male and female instrumental musicians. In: Principles of gender-specific medicine; 2017. p. 543–56.
11. Schuele SU, Lederman RJ. Occupational disorders in instrumental musicians. Med Probl Perform Art. 2004;19(3):123–9.
12. Lederman RJ. Neuromuscular and musculoskeletal problems in instrumental musicians. Muscle Nerve. 2003;27(5):549–61.
13. Lee HS, Park HY, Yoon JO, Kim JS, Chun JM, Aminata IW, et al. Musicians' medicine: musculoskeletal problems in string players. Clin Orthop Surg. 2013;5(3):155–60.
14. Lockwood AH. Medical problems of musicians. N Engl J Med. 1989;320(4):221–7.
15. Edwards RHT. Hypotheses of peripheral and central mechanisms underlying occupational muscle pain and injury. Eur Appl Physiol. 1988;57:275–81.
16. Thomas K, McCann P. Shoulder pain in musicians. Music Med. 2007;2(2):89–93.
17. Burnette JT, Ayoub MA. Cumulative trauma disorders. Pain Manag. 1989:196–209.
18. Lederman RJ, Calabrese LH. Overuse syndromes in instrumentalists. Med Prohl Perform Art. 1986;1(1):7–11.
19. Fry HJH. Overuse syndromes in instrumental musicians. Semin Neurol. 1989;9(2):136–45.
20. Bejjani FJ. Musicians occupational disorders. In: Proceedings of the International Conference for Health and the Musician. University of York; 1997.
21. Sheon RP. Repetitive strain injury. Diagnostic and treatment tips on six common problems. Postgrad Med. 1997;102(4):72–8.
22. Heming MJE. Occupational injuries suffered by classical musicians through overuse. Clin Chiropractic. 2004;7(2):55–66.
23. Fry HJH. Incidence of overuse syndrome in the symphony orchestra. Med Probl Perform Art. 1986;1(2):51–5.
24. Moore A, Wells R, Ranney D. Quantifying exposure in occupational manual tasks with cumulative trauma disorder potential. Ergonomics. 1991;34(12):1433–53.
25. Cohen R, Williams G. Impingement syndrome and rotator cuff disease as repetitive motion disorders. Clin Orthop. 1998;351:95–101.
26. Turner-Stokes K, Reid L. Three-dimensional motion analysis of upper limb movement in the bowing arm of string-playing musicians. Clin Biomech. 1999;14:426–33.
27. Rickert D, et al. A study of right shoulder injury in collegiate and professional orchestral cellists: an investigation using questionnaires and physical assessment. Med Probl Perform Art. 2012;27(2):65–73.
28. Moore M, DeHaan L, et al. Clinical assessment of shoulder impingement factors in violin and Viola players. Med Probl Perform Art. 2008;23:155–63.
29. Lederman RJ. Peripheral nerve disorders in instrumentalists. Ann Neurol. 1989;26:640–6.
30. Larsson LG, Baum J, Mudholkar GS, Kollia GD. Benefits and disadvantages of joint hypermobility among musicians. N Engl J Med. 1993;329(15):1079–82.
31. Bird H. Musculoskeletal problems encountered in musicians. Int Soc Study Tension Performance J. 1992;7:4–5.
32. Berque P, Gray H, McFadyen A. Playing-related musculoskeletal problems among professional orchestra musicians in Scotland: a prevalence study using a validated instrument, the musculoskeletal pain intensity and interference questionnaire for musicians (MPIIQM). Med Probl Perform Art. 2016;31:78–86.
33. MacIver H, Smyth G, Bird HA. Occupational disorders: non-specific forearm pain. Best Pract Res Clin Rheumatol. 2007;21:349–65.
34. Zaza C. Playing-related musculoskeletal disorders in musicians: a systematic review of incidence and prevalence. CMAJ. 1998;158(8):1019–25.

4 Dance

Gian Luigi Canata, Valentina Casale,
and Marcella Ioppolo

4.1 Introduction

Dance is a widely diffused performing art, including different styles and forms. Injuries are not rare, mostly related with overuse and faulty techniques.

Prevention is of paramount importance, mainly involving physical training and technical learning. An experienced medical staff may guarantee an optimal prevention and management of injuries.

4.2 History of Dance

Dance is a performing art consisting of selected sequences of movement. It has an aesthetic and symbolic value and may be categorized by its choreography, by types of movement performed, or by the historical period or place of origin. Dance may have different functions, such as social, competitive, ceremonial, martial, erotic, or sacred/liturgical meanings. Even several forms of athletics have a dance-like quality, like gymnastics, martial arts, figure skating, synchronized swimming, and many others. Early evidences of dance performances include 9000-year-old paintings, as well as Egyptian tomb paintings dated 3000 BC (Fig. 4.1).

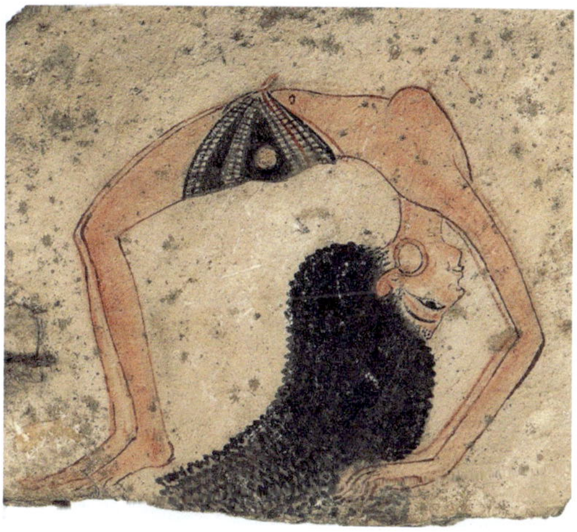

Fig. 4.1 Old Egyptian dancer (collection of the Egyptian Museum of Turin)

It may be said that before the birth of writing languages, dance was a fundamental method of handing down stories, and it had a main role during healing and religious rituals (Fig. 4.2).

G. L. Canata (✉) · V. Casale · M. Ioppolo
Koelliker Hospital, Centre of Sports Traumatology and Arthroscopic Surgery, Torino, Italy

H. Jones, A. Lukaszenko (eds.), *Injury Prevention and Care in Artistic Sports*,
https://doi.org/10.1007/978-3-032-18105-3_4

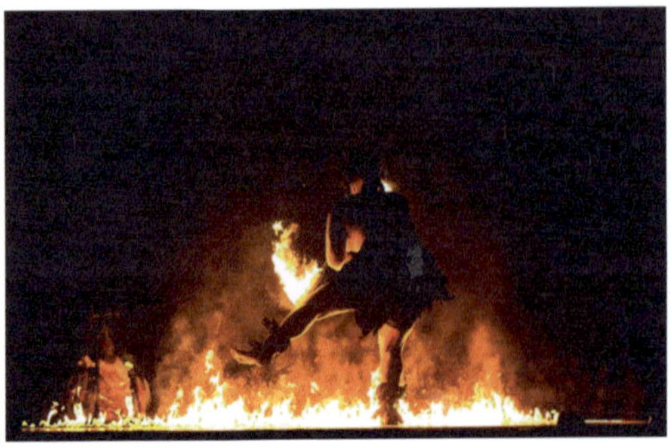

Fig. 4.2 Fire tribal dance

4.3 Different Kinds of Dances Like Different Kinds of Sports

A possible categorization of the existing dance styles includes modern dances (house dance, disco dance, punk dance), hip-hop and funk dance (breakdance, bounce, street jazz), ballroom dances (waltz, ballroom tango, mambo), African American and traditional jazz dances (Charleston, swing, boogie-woogie), worldwide dances and Latin dances (salsa, flamenco, tango, jive, capoeira, folk dances), and, finally, professional performance dances (ballet, contemporary dance, modern dance). Since the beginning of the twentieth century, competitive ballroom dances became popular with the name of dancesport. The first DanceSport World Championship took place in 1909, and its events were regulated at national and international levels, such as the World DanceSport Federation (WDSF). After a long campaign, the WDSF was recognized by the International Olympic Committee (IOC) in 1997.

Dance as a sport is a partnered activity with, normally, a male and female counterpart. Its disciplines include acrobatic rock 'n' roll, boogie-woogie, breakdance, disco dance, hip-hop, Latin dances (samba, cha-cha-cha, rumba, paso doble, and jive), rhythm (cha-cha, rumba, swing, bolero, and mambo), salsa, smooth (waltz, tango, foxtrot, and Viennese waltz), and handicapped dancer/sportive, which involves at least one athlete with a physical impairment affecting the lower limbs. The tango deserves a special mention, because it consists of a variety of styles that developed in different regions of Argentina and Uruguay, as well as in other areas around the globe. As a result, Argentine, Uruguayan, and ballroom tango include very different techniques, with consequent different physical demands. As several types of dance have evolved, so have the relative injuries. Because of that, dance medicine has kept evolving over the past 20 years, together with other professional figures and fields, such as choreographers, chiropractic, athletic training, acupuncture, and nutrition.

4.4 Epidemiology, Etiology, Typical, and Most Common Injuries in Dance

Many factors predispose to dance injuries, indeed, in addition to physical specific demands. Some examples are poor nutrition, eating disorders, stress, inadequate dance floor surfaces, wrong footwear, and much more. Physical complaints are a common aspect of dancers' everyday life. Still, only one third leads to a break from dance training; the rest is usually tolerated, ignored, or just considered as normal for a dancer's life. Injuries in dancers are very common; in fact, they are considered a natural, even necessary, part of participating in dance. However, acute injuries are relatively uncommon in dance. Chronic overuse causes the majority of time loss in dance and may predispose to acute traumas. Especially in ballet and modern dance, long hours of class, rehearsal, and performance typically begin at a young age, continue in the adolescent growth spurt, and involve repetitive moments like jumps. Furthermore, professional dancers may train up to 40 hours per week in addition to performances, and the high number of training hours and repetitions often results in a gradual wearing and tearing. Participation in dance is not intense and long lasting enough to improve substantially aerobic capacity, and low cardiorespiratory endurance has been proved to predispose to dance injuries. Traumatic injuries from acute stress are less common. Generally, they are caused by loss of balance during the performance: typical examples are ankle strains, hamstring strains, or patella dislocations. Overuse injuries are much more common, usually involving the lower extremities and lower back. Ballet movements often exceed anatomical limitations (e.g., turnout or pointe work), and modern dance requires high versatility (e.g., improvisation or inversions). These aspects lead to a higher susceptibility of dancers to injuries. Reported prevalence and incidence rates of musculoskeletal injuries among dancers show that dance is a high-risk activity, regardless of the style and level of participation. Among ballet dancers, the rates are particularly high, mostly affecting the lower extremity and the low back. Also, other forms of dance show high rates of injuries, such as jazz/contemporary dance, street dance, and tap/folk dance. Most injuries are due to overuse, with similar rates among males and females. Among professional dancers, however, the rate of traumatic injuries rises, especially in male dancers. There are no significant differences in different dancing levels, but it has been reported that low muscle strength levels in professional dancers are associated with an increased injury risk, and a reduced muscle strength may extend the recovery time. As reported by Meuffels et al. in Table 4.1, the lower extremity is the most frequent site affected [2].

Table 4.1 Dance injuries incidence per year among professional and pre-professional level dancers

Anatomic location	Professional dancers (%)	Dance students (%)
Neck	23	11
Shoulder	15	8
Arms/hands	10	5
Thoracic spine	11	7
Lumbar spine	47	42
Pelvis	15	16
Thigh	14	15
Lower leg	26	23
Knees	32	30
Ankles	42	30
Feet	33	21

Nevertheless, some dance styles involve the upper extremity too, as mentioned by Quin et al. in Table 4.2 [3].

4.4.1 Ankle and Foot Injuries

Foot and ankle injuries are commonly experienced among dancers. Focusing on ballet dancers, Vosseller et al. recently described the os trigonum syndrome (or posterior ankle impingement), the flexor hallucis longus (FHL) tenosynovitis, and the anterior ankle impingement as the most common problems in dancers [1]. In fact, the extreme plantarflexion involved in dancing and the consequent demands on the toe flexors induce or worsen these pathologies.

During some ballet figures, such as the "en pointe," a correct range of motion let the center of mass be aligned over the toe box, with the dorsum of the foot parallel to the tibia. If the talocrural joint plantar flexion is inadequate, a posterior ankle impingement may develop. This condition is described both in soft-tissue pathologies (as capsular impingement or the FHL tendinitis) and bony impingement (i.e., caused by the presence of an os trigonum or a Stieda process). Other frequent orthopedic situations in dancers are stress fractures and ankle sprains, with possible development of ankle instability, hallux valgus, and Morton's neuroma.

Table 4.2 Most common sites of injuries in different dance styles

Dance style	Most common sites of injury
Classical ballet	Foot and ankle
Contemporary/modern	Foot, ankle, lower back, and knee
Jazz	Foot, ankle, lower back, and knee
Ballroom	Foot and ankle
Flamenco	Foot
Pole dance	Wrist, elbow, and shoulder
Hip-hop/breakdancing	Wrist and elbow

4.4.2 Knee Injuries

Knee injuries are very common among dancers. The most frequent examples are patella femoral complaints, iliotibial band symptoms, patellar bursitis, and patellar tendinopathy. It must be reported that professional dancers show lower rates of such injuries because of a tough selection process, learning to deal with forced stressed positions or movements by hard training. ACL rupture has been reported to affect classical ballet dancers more often than contemporary ones; this is probably due to the higher number of jumps and landing in dehors, with the knee in a valgus position [2].

4.4.3 Hip Injuries

Several dance genres expose the hip joint to repetitive loading in extreme range of movements, and this may predispose to pain and injury. This trend has encouraged a higher interest for hip pathologies even for the better knowledge and less invasive treatments recently developed. The femoroacetabular subluxation or instability and the femoroacetabular impingement (FAI) are examples of the effects of the supra-physiological hip range of motion required in dance, especially in ballet.

Regardless of the hip joint anatomy, it has been reported that dancers experience FAI at the end points of the range of motion, even with a normal hip anatomy. The *ligamentum teres* tears are a further affection more frequently found among dancers than the general population: the ligamentum teres is in fact one of the hip stabilizers, and the microinstability of the hip caused by repeated extra ranges of motion may predispose to its tear. Interestingly, the prevalence of cam and pincer morphology among dancers is lower than in other athletes. It is unclear whether dancers do not simply develop these morphologies during adolescence, like other athletes do, or if it is due to a natural selection among dancers, because they limit the hip range of motion. Muscle lesions may be mentioned as the most frequent acute hip injuries. The most affected muscles are the inner thigh muscle at their attachment to the pubic bone, as well as the hamstrings close to their attachment at the ischial tuberosity.

In case of chronic overload, other frequent hip pathologies are:

- Iliopsoas syndrome.
- Snapping hip.
- Tendinitis at the great trochanter.
- Piriformis syndrome.
- Hip impingement.
- Labral tears.
- Osteoarthritis.

4.4.4 Lower-Back Injuries

Contemporary and ballet dancers show a high prevalence of low-back pain, mostly associated with activity modifications, care seeking, and medication use.

Furthermore, keeping alternate full flexion and extension movements may predispose to the development of spinal pathologies such as spondylolysis.

4.4.5 Upper-Extremity Injuries

Because dance is mainly weightbearing with the lower extremity, the reported rates of upper-extremity injuries have always been low.

Nevertheless, demands for the upper extremities have recently increased in some choreographic figures, such as floor work, movements requiring support of the body by the arms, and women partnering other women or man. Breakdancing is the most high-demanding discipline on upper extremities, especially on the hands, wrist, shoulder, and neck. Furthermore, modern dance may require contact improvisation, with consequent additional stress to the upper extremity. Also jazz dance includes acrobatic figures of hip-hop and breakdancing, thus causing high stresses on upper extremities. Recently, pole dance has become increasingly popular: it is another example of high-demanding discipline on the upper extremity, requiring a focus on the range of motion and strength of the core, the upper body, and the upper limbs.

When approaching a dance injury, the first question to be made should be: "Which technical fault has led to this injury?" The most common causes are intrinsic indeed: not all dancers are anatomically predisposed to specific dance disciplines.

Therefore, it is fundamental to realize as soon as possible the exact possible anatomical limitations, so that the dancer may learn how to work within his/her physical range, without going beyond his/her physical potential. Professional dancers should ideally present loose joints, turnout of the leg, slight knee hyperextension, and adequate flexion of the ankle and the foot.

Dance performance requires support from enhanced physiological capabilities, including flexibility, muscular strength, power, and endurance. The physiological requirements are a large reserve of power for explosive jumps and high elevation or during the act of lift, as well as muscular endurance, which occurs when a relatively high-power output is maintained.

Contributing risk factors to dance injuries are [4]:

- Improper training.
- Faulty technique, in particular considering the jump landing technique: a higher ground reaction force and impulse may predispose to patella tendinopathy; also, the repetition of double heel strike may predispose to the development of shin splints.
- Previous injury.
- Anthropometrics aspects (such as low body mass index, low adiposity, or increased thigh circumference).
- Poor aerobic capacity.
- Lower-extremity altered alignment (such as sacrum inclination angle during turnout lower than 30°, leading to possible development of lumbosacral pain).
- Structural deformity of the foot.
- Psychological factors (such as poor coping skills).
- Environmental hazard (such as hard floors).
- Biomechanical imbalance.

4.5 Diagnosis

The clinical and radiographic evaluation is the same used in case of sports trauma. Specifically, the clinician should pay attention to the dance movement that has caused the injury; the dancers should be asked to reply it, in order to better understand the dynamic of the trauma. It is also paramount to always consider the dance style practiced and its specific technical demands, because it will help better understand and management the specific cases.

4.6 Medical Treatment

The first fundamental aspect to consider is the patient's artistic background, his/her technique and style, in order to better understand the mechanism of injury and to successfully prevent re-injury. The role of a company physiotherapist is unique, to screen, guide, and treat injuries.

Beside this, a strict collaboration with orthopedic surgeons is essential to promptly address urgent traumatic lesions, as well as to assess when an overuse injury requires surgery [2]. The basis of any treatment, regardless of the site and the entity of injury, is to modify the movement pattern that has led to the pathogenesis of the problem. Basically, the technique must be deeply understood and correctly applied. When surgery is the treatment of choice, the company team should council and inform the dancers of all the pros and cons of operative treatment: dancers in fact need to perform and get back on stage as quickly and safely as possible. Surgery is usually reserved to cases of traumatic overuse injuries not manageable with conservative treatment.

4.7 Physiotherapy

In almost every dance style, the lower extremity undergoes high stresses, especially considering the ankle and the foot. For this reason, it is paramount for a good rehabilitation and an effective return to dance to understand and practice some specific exercises. For example, classic ballet dancers need to stretch and strengthen both the feet arch and the toe extensors muscles. To do this, some specific training exercises are usually recommended, such as those showed in Fig. 4.3.

Considering every kind of dance instead, the pelvic alignment is of great importance among dancers, and its deficit often results in a faulty technique and higher risks of injury.

The neutral pelvis is a position defined by the anterior superior iliac spine and pubic bone being on the same plane; its most common deviations are the anterior tilt or the posterior tilt.

Among dancers, the anterior pelvic tilt is frequently seen, and it may be associated to tight hip flexors and low-back pain. To achieve a proper alignment for an aesthetic line and form, and to effectively execute complex movement patterns, the Pilates method has been recently adopted among dancers during both everyday training and the recovery regimen after injury (Figs. 4.4, 4.5, 4.6, 4.7, 4.8, and 4.9).

Pilates is a distinctive system of physical and mental conditioning; it is designed to strengthen and balance the body, stabilizing the core musculature, including abdominals, gluteus, and paravertebral muscles, and then it proceeds through a controlled range of motion. In response to a small number of repetition (usually no more than ten), the body is regularly exposed to new muscular and kinesthetic demands, coordinating breathing and precise placement, and requiring constant concentration.

The key elements of Pilates are:

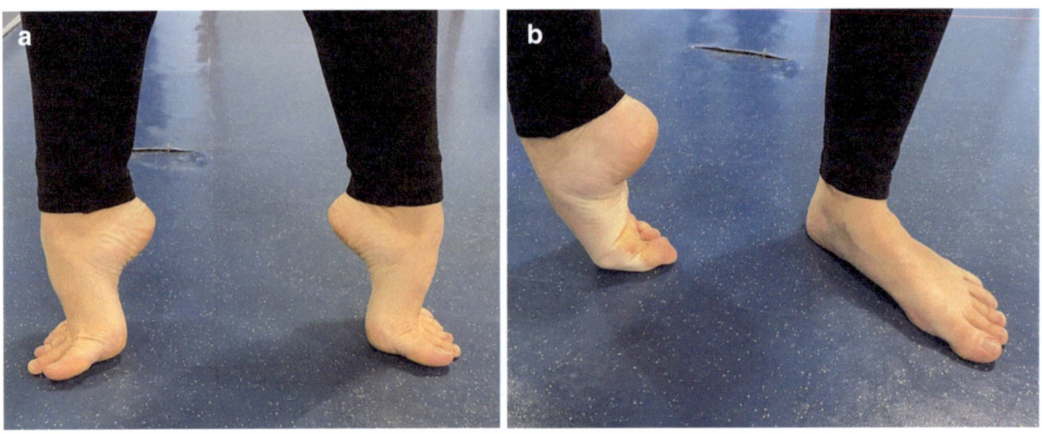

Fig. 4.3 (**a**) *Relevé* figure, reaching a bilateral demi pointe with lengthened toes (it stretches the foot arch). (**b**) Rising to *pointe* one foot at a time (it stretches the toe extensor foot muscles)

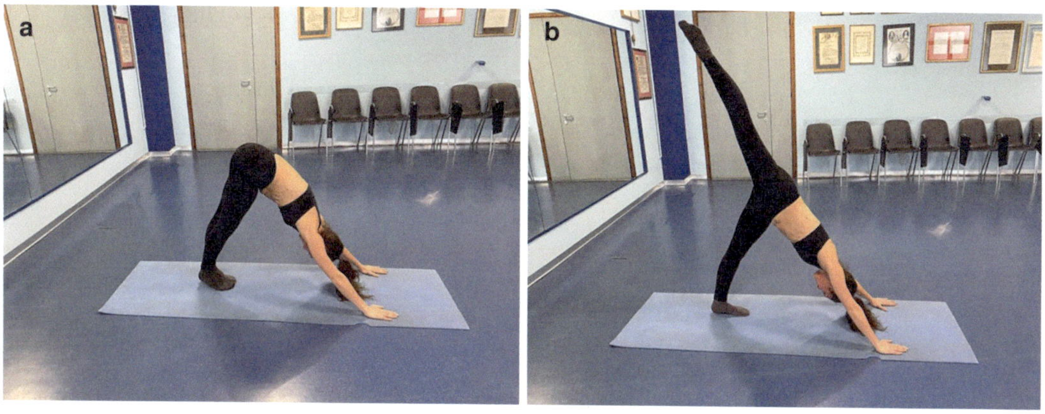

Fig. 4.4 (**a**) Downward-facing dog pose (it stretches the shoulders, hamstrings, calves, arches, and hands and strengthens the arms and legs). (**b**) Three-legged downward dog pose (over the benefits of the downward-facing dog, it also stretches the inner and outer hip)

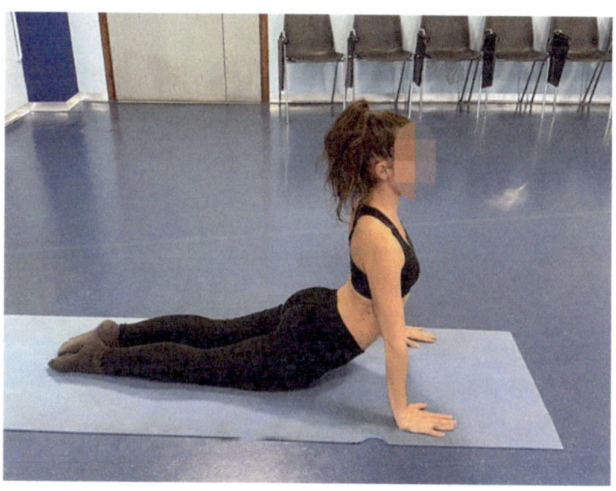

Fig. 4.5 Upward-facing dog pose (it stretches the chest and lungs, shoulder, and abdomen and strengthens the spine, arms, and wrists)

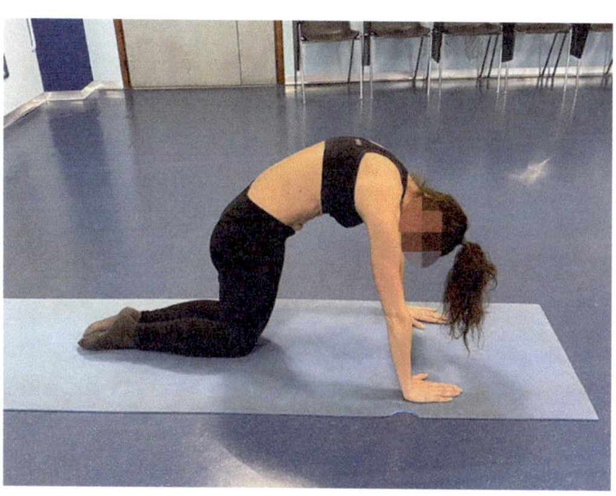

Fig. 4.6 Cat pose—inspiration (it stretches the hips, abdomen, and back and strengthens the spine and the neck during inspiration)

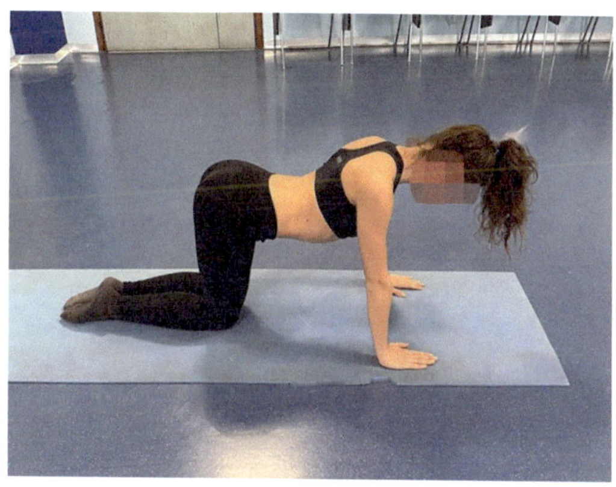

Fig. 4.7 Cow pose—expiration (same benefits of the cat pose but during expiration)

- Concentration: cognitive attention is required to perform every exercise.
- Centering through tightening the muscular center of the body, between the pelvic floor and ribcage during exercises.
- Control through the management of posture and movement during the exercises.
- Precision.
- Flow: a smooth transition within the exercises is recommended.
- Breath: moving air into and out of the lungs in coordination with exercise.

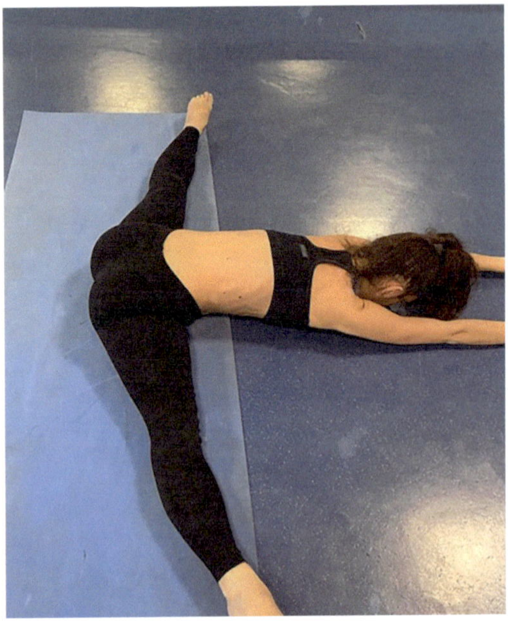

Fig. 4.8 Wide angle forward fold (it stretches and strengthens the hamstrings, calves, hips, low back, and spine while stretching the shoulders, wrists, forearms, and upper back too)

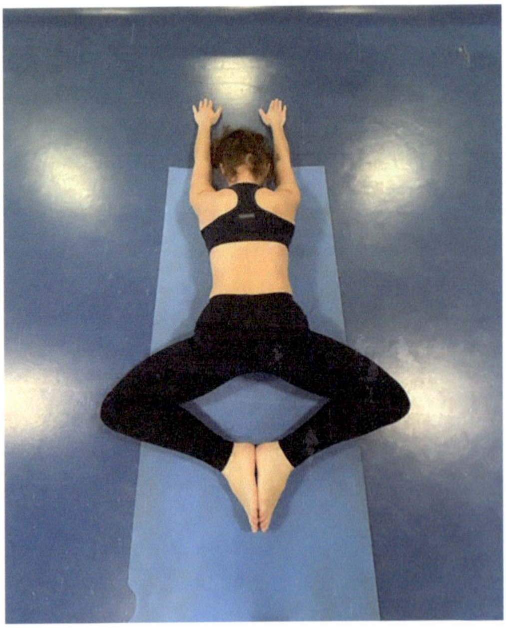

Fig. 4.9 Frog pose (it opens the hip joints, improves abduction, and strengthens the lower back)

4.8 Return to Performance

The goal of dance rehabilitation is to prepare the athlete to a successful return to previous level of performance, identifying the cause of injury and minimizing at the same time the risk of reinjury. Dance-specific rehabilitation is fundamental to reaching the best possible outcomes. Addressing physical function is not the only aspect to deal with. In dance, the nature of choreography and the specific roles can vary considerably. For these reasons, return to stage needs to be carefully evaluated from the dancer with the help of the artistic, clinical, and conditioning staff. The artistic staff should clarify the likely physical demands in upcoming rehearsal and performance roles, and the dancer's perspectives should be clearly understood. From a clinical point of view, in the absence of pre-season baseline data, a limb symmetry testing may provide a useful criterion for injuries to lower and upper extremities.

In particular, the following aspects should be considered and evaluated:

- Functional movement testing to assess movement skills and neuromuscular control.
- Joints range of motion (ROM), especially in the lower extremities.
- Balance/proprioception through some tests like the star excursion balance test (SEBT) or the single-leg test.
- Muscle power by jumping analysis (observing height, symmetry, distance on single hop and repeated hops, crossovers, speed over distance).
- Muscle strength of the knee and sagittal motion of the ankle.

Understanding the functional requirements of dance and the complexity of several figures is of paramount importance for returning to performance. For example, when landing from specific jumping figures such as pliè and demi-pliè, returning the heel to the ground requires a systematic eccentric control sequence, which starts from the foot, and then the knee is unlocked from an initial straight position, but at the same time, the lowering is regulated by the glutes and the posterior chain. Evaluating the whole sequence is very difficult by using objective measurements only. For this reason, there are tests that grade the quality of the control through the foot, then the knees, and hips, often with the use of a metronome, also evaluating the symmetry between the affected and the unaffected sides. Dance often involves prolonged bouts of high-intensity intervals against longer work of a lower intensity. For a strength and power endurance assessment, a useful test evaluates repeated strength (repeated lifts or rises) and power drills (jump box plyometric drills) with short recovery. Assessing chronic training load is also important to establish whether the dancer may return to a performance period, and not just to a single show.

4.9 Prevention

The prevention of dance-related injuries is mandatory. It may basically consist in:

- Screening of dancer's physical and psychological attributes, prior injuries, and planned dance activity.
- Physical training encouragement, with special attention to the core and the musculature specific demanding of the genre.
- Proper nutrition and rest, reducing the fatigue.
- Provision of specialized healthcare services for risk assessment, injury management, and injury reduction.

The main purpose is to determine whether there are any anatomical areas that may cause technical difficulties or injury either during training or later in a professional career; when assessing adults, it is helpful to identify any issue correlated to the type of dance practiced. Since some physical aspects may occasionally preclude any satisfactory participation in dance, for example, classical ballet, these examinations may guide a young dancer along the right lines, maybe choosing a different type of dance.

The orthopedic surgeon should always evaluate if there is any physical problem calling for an outright rejection for dance practice (such as an established spondylolisthesis) or those characteristics potentially dangerous in the future.

To carefully analyze all these aspects, some authors have proposed a card to be submitted to all dancers, whatever discipline or level is practiced (Table 4.3).

Since the main cause of dance injury is faulty technique, conversely a good technique prevents the risks of incurring injuries. A correct muscle balance is as important as muscle strength, especially for movement control. Over-bulky muscles may be in fact a disadvantage to the dancer due to changes in the center of gravity of the body, which lead to instability during dance.

Furthermore, the overemphasis often placed on building up the quadriceps in the thigh may lead to neglecting other primary muscle groups of the same region like the adductors, the hamstrings, and the gluteals.

Five main areas of attention for preventing dance injuries have been proposed:

- Warming-up and training (focusing on muscular strength, power, plyometrics, agility, balance, joint stability, and dance-specific technique).
- Equipment (including footwear and surfaces).
- Regulatory aspects, such as rules and regulations governing dance.
- Self-care prevention.
- Treatment methods.

Table 4.3 Assessment card for dancers' physical evaluation according to Howse and McCormack

ORTHOPAEDIC ASSESSMENT		
Name................................. Age....................................... Height.................. BMI......................................		Date of birth............. Weight....................
Neck	ROM:	Tight trapezius:
Shoulder girdle	Asymmetry: Winged scapulae: Elbows:	Glenohumeral joint range: Wrists:
Pelvis	Level:	Asymmetry:
Spine	Scoliosis: Thoracic spine flex: Thoracic spine rotation: Lumbar spine flex: Lumbar spine side flex: General view:	Kyphosis: Thoracic spine extension: Thoracic spine side flex: Lumbar spineextend:
Lower limb	R Hamstrings: R Achilles:	L Hamstrings: L Achilles:
Knees	Hyperextension: Patellae:	Genu valgus: Tibial bow:
Foot	Pointe: R L Ankle: R L Rt big toe extension: Lesser toes: R midtarsal: R subtalar:	Metatarsus: R L Lt big toe extension: Metatarsals: L midtarsal: L subtalar:
Hips	Rotation extended: R ER: R IR: L ER: L IR: Rotation flexed: R ER: R IR: L ER: L IR:	
General	Past injury Operations: Investigations:	Beighton (joint hypermobility): Growth: General health:
Other comments		
Examiner		Date

4.10 Summary

Dance is a widely diffused performing art, including different styles and performing mechanisms. Injuries are mostly related with overuse and faulty techniques. Prevention is of huge importance, with adequate protocols and systematic exercises, mainly involving physical training and technical learning. An experienced medical staff, close to the performers, may guarantee an optimal prevention and management of injuries.

References

1. Vosseller JT, Dennis ER, Bronner S. Ankle injuries in dancers. J Am Acad Orthop Surg. 2019;27:582–9.
2. Meuffels DE, Agricola R, Calder J. Dance orthopaedics ballet injuries and when to perform surgical treatment. In: Kerkhoffs GMMJ, et al., editors. ESSKA instructional course lecture: Glasgow 2018. Springer; 2018. p. 343–53.
3. Quin E, Rafferty S, Tomlinson C. Dance injury pattern. In: Quin E, et al., editors. Safe dance practice. Human Kinetics; 2015. p. 179–82.
4. Kenny SJ, Whittaker JL, Emery CA. Risk factors for musculoskeletal injury in preprofessional dancers: a systematic review. Br J Sports Med. 2016;50(16):997–1003.

5 Bull's Performance

Henrique Jones

5.1 Introduction

> There are only three sports: mountain climbing, bull fighting and motor racing, all the rest are merely games. –Ernest Hemingway

Bullfights are traditional spectacles of Spain, Portugal, some places in the south of France and some America Latina countries as Mexico, Colombia, Ecuador, Venezuela and Peru. In the USA, there is the rodeo tradition and Portuguese-style bullfighting in California. Many supporters of bullfighting do believe deeply that this tradition is ingrained and is an important part of their national cultures. Bullfighting is seen as a symbol of *Spanish culture*, and in Spain, it is called "El Festival Nacional" (National Festival). The aesthetic of bullfighting is based on the interaction of the man and the bull (Fig. 5.1).

Rather than a competitive sport [1], bullfighting is more of a ritual of ancient origin, which is judged by bullfighting fans based on artistic impression and command, Ernest Hemingway said in his 1932 non-fiction book *Death in the Afternoon* (Fig. 5.2).

"Bullfighting is the only art in which the artist is in danger of death and in which the degree of brilliance in the performance is left to the fighter's honour [2]." Those who oppose bullfighting maintain that the practice is a cowardly, sadistic tradition of torturing, humiliating and killing a bull amidst pomp and pageantry. Supporters of bullfights claim they respect the bulls who live better, and longer, than other cattle and that bullfighting is a secular tradition and form of art. Its critics regard the bullfight as a demonstration of style, technique and courage by its participants and as a demonstra-

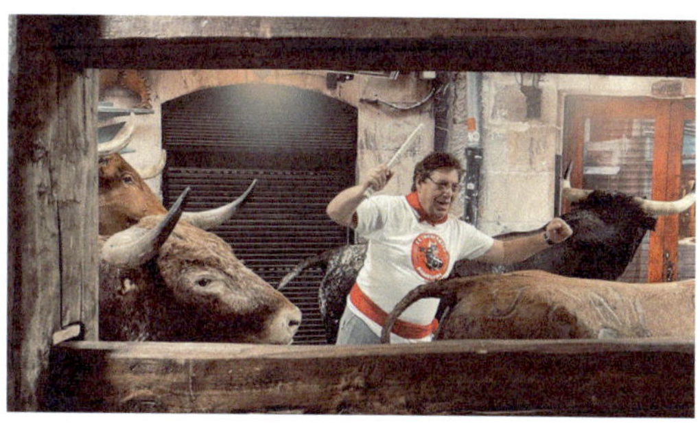

Fig. 5.1 Bull runners in Pamplona

H. Jones (✉)
Hospital da Luz, Setúbal Orthopedic Surgery and Sports Medicine, Montijo Orthopedic Sports Med Clinic, Setubal, Portugal

H. Jones, A. Lukaszenko (eds.), *Injury Prevention and Care in Artistic Sports*,
https://doi.org/10.1007/978-3-032-18105-3_5

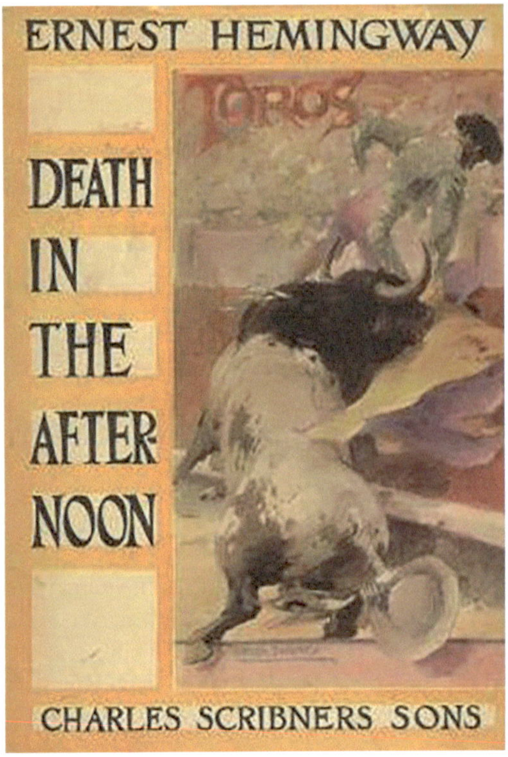

Fig. 5.2 Death in the afternoon

tion of cruelty and cowardice. While there is usually no doubt about the outcome, the bull is viewed by bullfighting supporters as a worthy adversary, deserving of respect in its own right. Bulfighting will always be a controverse topic regarding the definition as sport, art, culture or barbarian. Bulfighting could simply mean running`s or bull rodeos and all modalities involve specific injuries (Fig. 5.1) or bull rodeos, the reality is that this kind of "exhibitions" exists and they involve specific injuries that must be recognize by medical doctors, nurses and physios in order to establish appropriate treatment and prevention strategies.

5.2 History and Tradition in Most Important Bullfighting Countries

5.2.1 Bullfighting in Spain

Bullfighting is an iconic tradition in Spain and one of the defining cultural characteristics of this Iberian country. Spanish bullfighting was first brought to the attention of the Western world in Ernest Hemingway's novel, *A Sun Also Rises*. It remains a curious attraction for many travellers in Spain, despite the ongoing disputes between moral activists and die-hard bullfighting followers. Bullfighting in Spain traces its origins to AD 711, with the first official bullfight being held in honour of the coronation of King Alfonso VIII. Once part of the Roman Empire, Spain owes its bullfighting tradition in part to gladiator games. At first, bullfighting was done on horseback and was reserved for Spanish aristocracy, but King Felipe V ended this trend because he believed it was in poor taste for nobles to practice such a bloody sport. Commoners continued to develop bullfighting on foot with smaller weapons. The art of dodging and stabbing the bull grew into its present form around 1724, and bullfighters today still cling to a traditionally strict code of conduct. The oldest bullring in Spain is located in the southern town of Ronda, but cities like Madrid, Seville and Pamplona also have a rich bullfighting legacy and some of the largest rings in the world. This "Fiesta" could not exist without the wild bull (*Toro bravo*), a species of bull of an archaeal race that is only conserved in Spain. Formerly, this bull's forebears, the primitive urus, were spread out over wide parts of the world. Many civilizations revered to them. The bull cults at the Greek island Crete is quite well known. The first recorded bullfight may be the Epic of Gilgamesh, which describes a scene in which Gilgamesh and Enkidu fought and killed the Bull of Heaven. The Bible reports on sacrifices of bulls in honour to the divine justice. Also in the religious ceremonies of Iberian tribes, living in Spain, in prehistorical times, bulls played an important part in those ceremonies. While the religious cults to the bull goes back to Iberians, it was the Greek and Roman influence that converted it into a spectacle.

During the Middle Ages, it was a diversion for the aristocracy fighting bulls on horse's back. In the eighteenth century, this tradition was more or less abandoned, and the poorer population invented the bullfight by foot. Francisco Romero was a key figure in laying the rules for that new sport.

5.2.2 Bullfighting in Mexico

Mexico has outlawed bullfighting twice in its history, but the sport is currently legal. Though bullfighting is a 500-year-old tradition, many Mexicans view it as cruel and unnecessary, and they push for its abolition, even participating in anti-bullfighting protests. Animal rights activists argue that while the objective of the sport is to kill the bull quickly and cleanly, that's often not the actual outcome, as it can take a matador several attempts to successfully kill the animal with a sword.

5.2.3 American Bullfighting

Freestyle bullfighting has always been a crowd favourite at rodeos and special events. In the last decade, the focus has been on the bull riders and the bulls with the unsung heroes going without events that will showcase their "tools of the trade" and unmatched skills. This is truly man against beast, with our modern-day gladiators risking everything in a 90-s match. The rodeo athletes are judged on how well they manoeuvre around a Mexican fighting bull. Death-defying feats are attempted, such as jumping over a bull and staying within inches of the bull's head. Freestyle bullfighting is a style of bullfighting developed in American rodeo. The style was developed by the rodeo clowns who protect bull riders from being trampled or gored by an angry bull. Freestyle bullfighting is a 70-s competition in which the bullfighter (rodeo clown) avoids the bull by means of dodging, jumping and use of a barrel.

A distinct type of bloodless bullfighting is practised in California's Central Valley. In this historically Portuguese-settled area, a form of bullfight has developed in which the bull is taunted by a matador, but the lances are tipped with Velcro and aimed at Velcro patches secured to the bull's shoulder.

5.2.4 Portuguese Bullfighting

Bullfights originated from worshipping practices and from the preparation of nobleman and horses for war. The origins of these practices cannot be dated back in time, but they exist in Portugal since the country was founded on the twelfth century. The Portuguese equestrian bullfighting is based on the developments of high school, presenting artistic and aristocratic features. From the eighteenth century on, bullfighting became more artistic, and it is nowadays considered performative art. In Portuguese bullfighting, there are bullfighters (*cavaleiros*) on horseback and a group of eight men (forcados) that grab the bull barehanded, and the bull is not killed at the end of the performance.

5.3 Frequent Injuries in Bullfighting

5.3.1 Statistics

Bullfighting is a "supremely dangerous art", says Garry Marvin, professor of human-animal studies at Roehampton University. "If a normal person got into the ring with a fighting bull, I'd expect them to be severely gored or dead in a few moments." Matadors are highly skilled, however, and may go several seasons without injury. What do the figures say? Bullfighting in Spain is run by the Ministry of Education, Culture and Sport—but surprisingly, no statistics on injuries are kept. Some unofficial figures do exist, however. In the 2013 season, 31 matadors received horn wounds, according to http://datoros.com. Some were minor and some life-threatening. Aside from the matadors themselves, 16 of their assistants were injured—the assistants usually include "picadors" on horseback, "banderilleros" on foot and a sword page (Table 5.1). These 47 injuries occur red during a total of 661 bullfights in Spain in

Table 5.1 Injury registration in Plaza Mexico

Injury	Numbers
Soft tissue injuries (major, requiring operative debridement)	57
Upper extremity	5
Lower extremity	52
Vascular injuries (requiring operative intervention)	5
Femoral vein	1
Femoral artery	4
Open fractures	1
Upper extremity	0
Lower extremity	1
Closed fractures	4
Upper extremity	4
Lower extremity	0
Articular dislocations	4
Shoulder	4
Total	91

2013 (the ministry does count how many bullfights take place). The profession is less perilous than it was, thanks to advances in medicine and the presence of specialist surgeons on standby to operate in the bullring nursery whenever it is needed. The last Spanish matador to die was Jose Cubero "El Yiyo" Sanchez in 1985. Alexander Fiske-Harrison, author of *Into The Arena: The World of the Spanish Bullfight*, cites records showing that 533 professional bullfighters have been killed in Spain since 1700. However, the records may be incomplete, he says, as bullfighting has only been regulated for 100 years.

5.4 The Bullfighter's Injury Patterns

5.4.1 Types of Injuries

Injury and death are inherent to the nature of bullfighting. The lack of training of amateur bullfighters might pose an additional threat in this group for serious injuries to occur. Since the bull and bullfighter are in unique, repetitive positions to each other, certain body sites of the bullfighter are at an increased risk of being injured. Udo Rudloff et al. aimed to study these mechanisms and types of injuries caused by organized bullfighting during a 10-year period at the second-largest bullfight arena of Mexico (Table 5.1).

This finding of disproportionally high incidence of injuries to the inguinal and perineal area, with a significant likelihood of associated injuries to the femoral vessels, supports the concept that these injuries follow a specific pattern due to the inherent nature of bullfighting. The height of the attacking bull's horns at the level of the bullfighter's waist, rotation of the gored and air-lifted bullfighter causing large wound cavities and the exposed perineal and genital areas to the passing bull's horn are examples of mechanisms of injuries unique to the occupation of bullfighters. Attempts to further reduce injuries during bullfighting should focus on the one side on thorough training of the toreros (Fig. 5.3).

5.4.2 Type of Injuries Produced in Popular Spectacles Involving Bulls

In this type of events, amateur bullfighters are involved, and open horn wounds are common. Most of them are located in the perineal area (also known as impalement injuries), which are due to run in front of the bull and being gored (Fig. 5.4). "Recordadores," people that jump over and fake the bulls, are skilled people exposed to severe injuries.

R. M. Cozcolluela Cabrejas et al. wrote an interesting paper with a retrospective analysis of patients who received urgent assistance in the hospital with pathology related to bulls for 10 years, between 2006 and 2015. In this paper, the injury rate was much higher in amateurs than professionals, meaning that professional skills and preparation were the most important reason for this difference (Fig. 5.5).

5.4.2.1 Type of Injuries Reported

Injuries are classified in bullfighters as open wounds (59), blunt trauma (secondary to high-energy trauma) (33) and mixed in patients with external injuries being associated to that one (11). The overall locations of the lesions were as follows: 32 located at the thigh, 21 at the leg, 14 at perineum, 8 at abdominal and 7 at thoracic region, 6 at the arms, 5 at the brain and craniofacial and 6 at the spine. Bull horn wounds were

Fig. 5.3 Incidence of injuries in bullfighter participants: young bullfighters (*novillero*) are the most injured between all

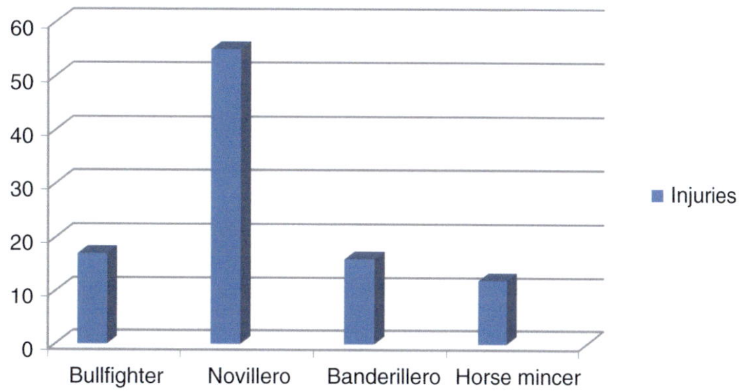

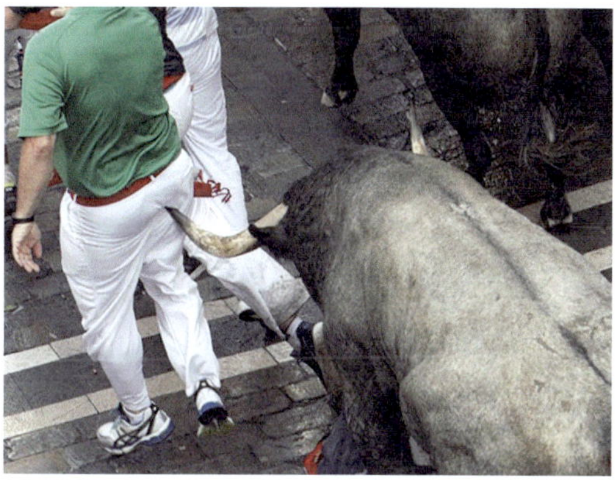

Fig. 5.4 Impalement injuries caused by bull horns. (Courtesy Iñaki Vergara)

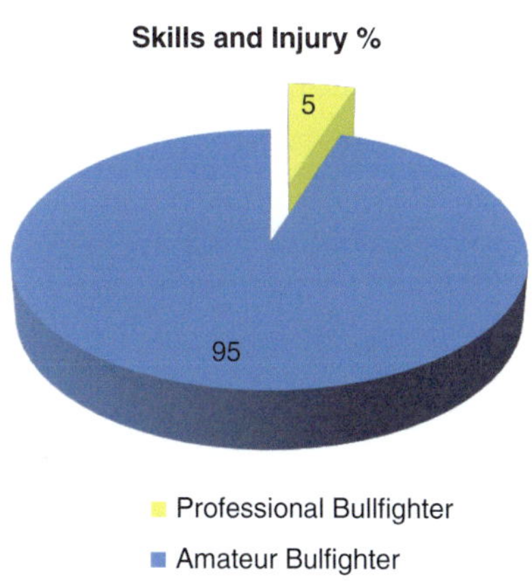

Fig. 5.5 Relation between professional and amateur bullfighters

more frequently located in the lower extremities and perineum. Blunt trauma lesions affected more frequently the thorax, brain, facial bones and spine. Surgical debridement was the most frequent treatment applied (Fig. 5.6). These injuries caused during popular bullfighting festivities in which amateur bullfighters participate are different from those that occur in professional bullfighting, although they are equally dangerous. Due to the complexity of the injuries, patients should be treated as polytrauma cases [3].

5.4.3 The Portuguese Reality

In Portugal, the traditional bullfighting involves horsemen (*cavaleiro*) (Fig. 5.7) and bull catchers (*forcados*) (Fig. 5.8).

Even though there is no statistics in "Forcados" injury incidence and pattern, important injuries are very frequent in those people: fractures of the lower limbs (including foot fractures by bull's paw) (Fig. 5.9), shoulder dislocation, rib fractures, knee multi-ligament injuries (Fig. 5.10), raquis fractures, face and skull injuries and muscle and tendon injuries. Perforate wounds and visceral involvement are present, but rare, due to the fact that the horns of the bull are protected by special scaffold.

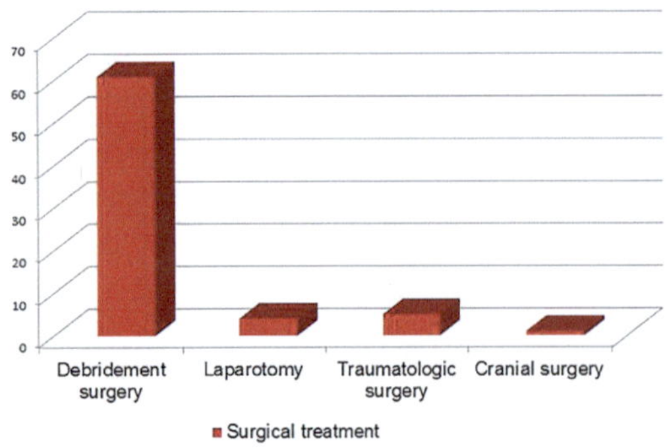

Fig. 5.6 Surgical treatment applied to injured bullfighters

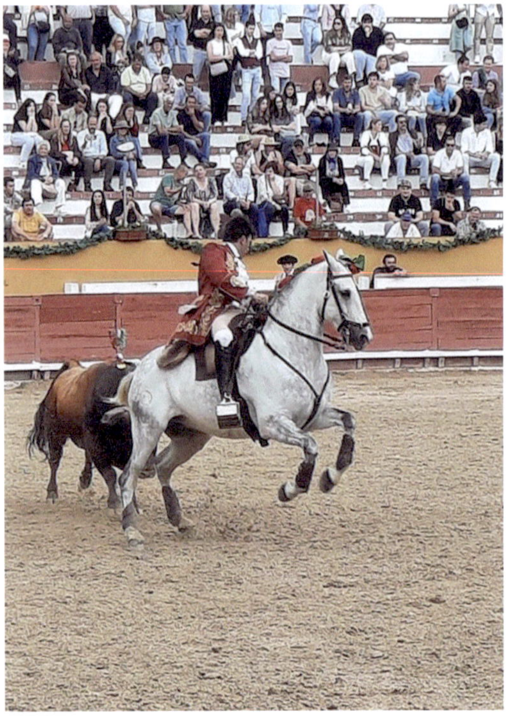

Fig. 5.7 Horseman bullfighter (*cavaleiro*)

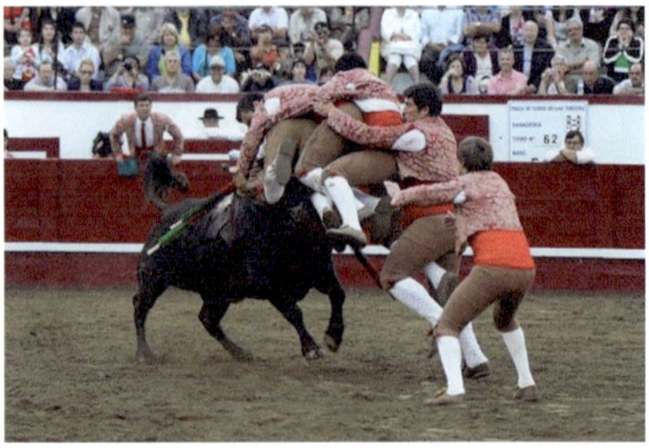

Fig. 5.8 Bull catchers (*forcados*)

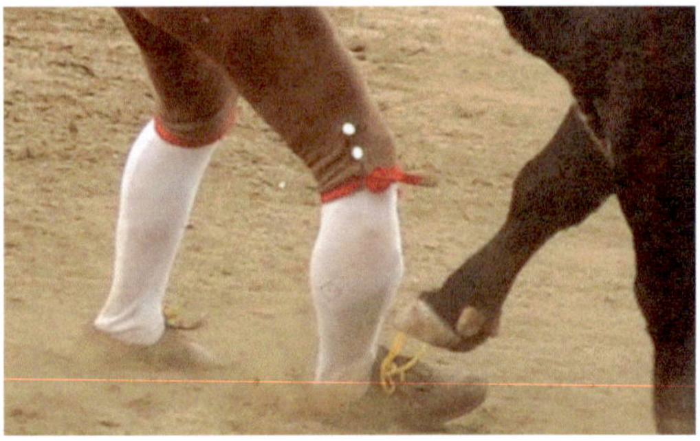

Fig. 5.9 Bull paw trauma

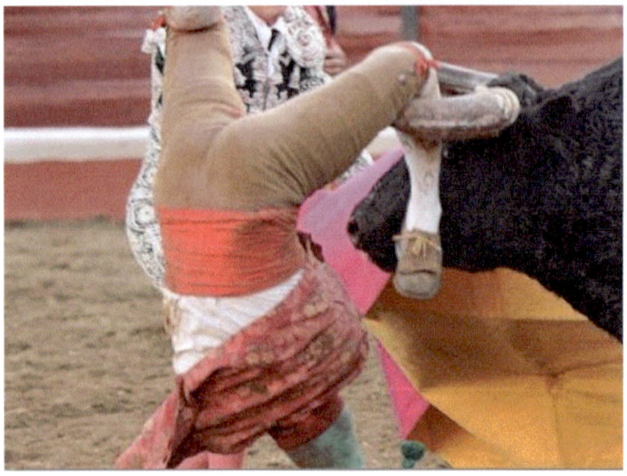

Fig. 5.10 Multi-ligament injury of the left knee caused by bull impact. (Courtesy Dr. Pedro Pessoa)

5.5 Prevention Generalities

5.5.1 Protection Devises

5.5.1.1 Equipment

Preventive equipment should be expected, to be improved, and used, to prevent the most severe injuries in bullfighters. As of the moment, there are some protective devices that pretend to minimize the importance of most frequent injuries. Bullfighter clothes have special characteristics respecting traditional patterns to prevent injuries by wearing tight, smooth trousers on which the horns of the bull more easily slide away. "Picadores" use special protection boots, and horses are protected by a very resistant coverage all over their bodies (Fig. 5.11a). Rodeo body, and head, protections and functional tapping are frequently used (Fig. 5.11b, c).

5.5.1.2 Training

Since many years ago, bullfighter training became a reality and a routine practice to adapt performance demands.

Bullfighters need to develop agility, strength, neuromuscular control, aerobic condition and mental capacity. It's important to be in peak physical shape if you want to become someone acting with bulls.

5.5.1.3 Aerobic and Mental Training

Strive to be able to engage in vigorous aerobic activity for a prolonged period of time. Building stamina can be achieved by working in the gym and using equipment like elliptical machines, treadmills and stationary bikes (Fig. 5.12). Running and jogging are also options.

As in other sports, chest strap Bluetooth monitoring of bullfighters is frequently used to control heart behaviour (Fig. 5.13).

5.5.1.4 Strength Training

Muscle building is fundamental by weightlifting and other forms of weight training. Strength training should include the upper and lower body in order to keep a good performance and a good attitude against unexpected situations. Practicing to improve balance and agility is also fundamental. Exercise programmes like CrossFit, triathlon training and other forms of exercise that engage multiple muscle groups and skill sets are encouraged.

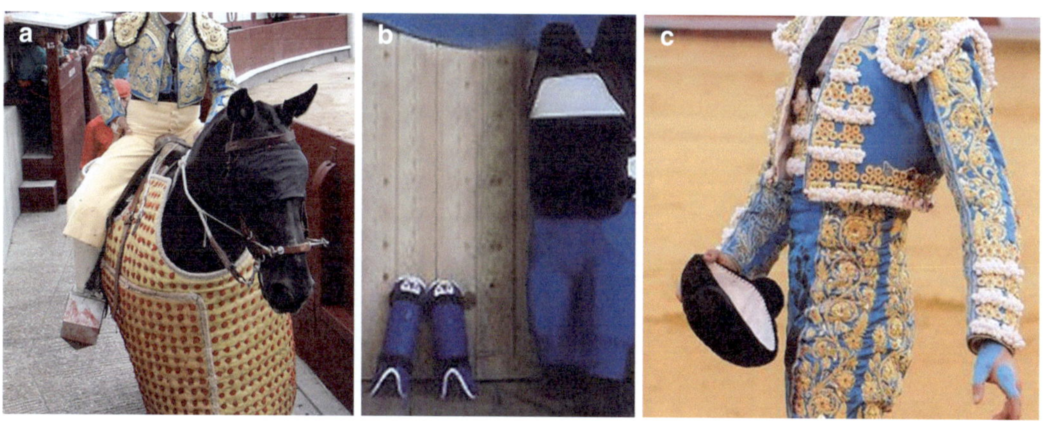

Fig. 5.11 Protective equipment. (**a**) Picador boots. (**b**) Rodeo equipment. (**c**) Functional tapping in the hand

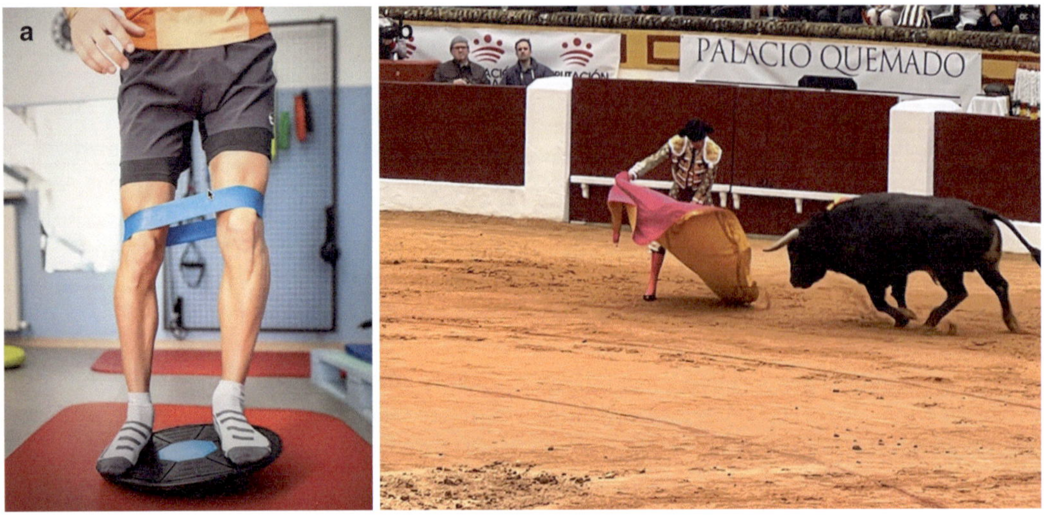

Fig. 5.12 Bullfighter (**a**) at training and (**b**) at the arena

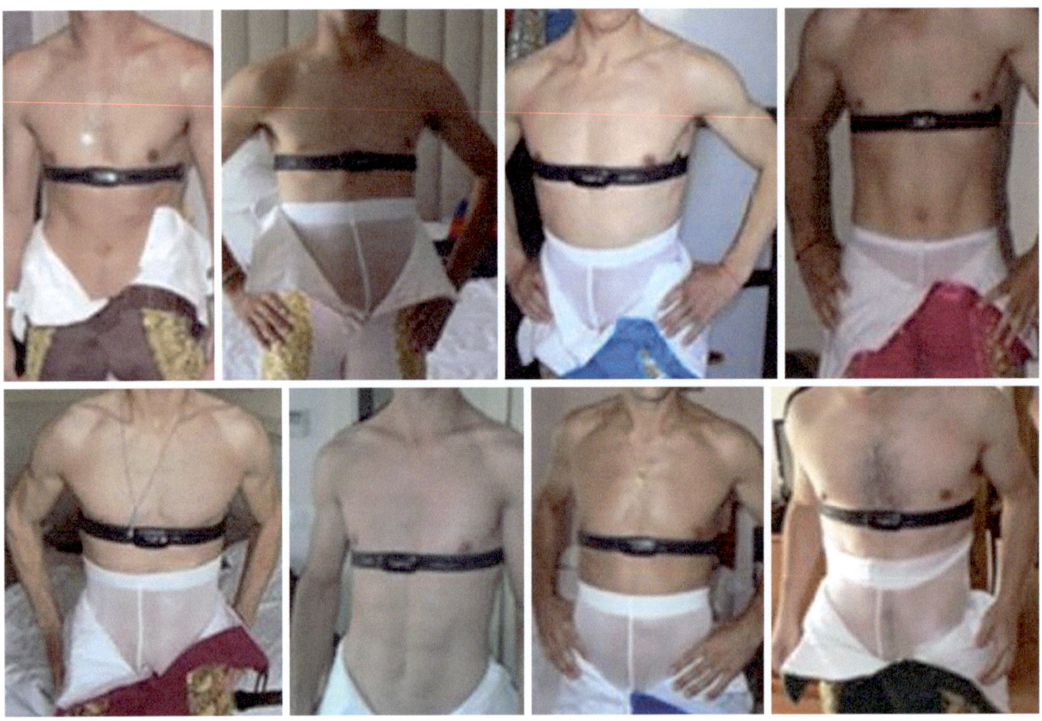

Fig. 5.13 Several bullfighters using heart rate monitoring

5.6 Specific Prevention Injury Programme for Bullfighters

Considering the high demands of bullfighting performers, a systematic injury prevention programme is highly important for these professionals. Similar to other sports that adapted the FIFA 11+ as the preferential prevention programme, with sport-specific modifications, it is important that it could serve as a model programme to these professional bullfighters.

The FIFA 11+ injury prevention programme was developed in 2006 to address this matter, under the leadership of the FIFA Medical Assessment and Research Centre and in collaboration with the Oslo Sports Trauma Research Centre and the Santa Monica Orthopaedic and Sports Medicine Centre. The programme comprises a complete warm-up procedure aimed at injury prevention in soccer players. It includes 15 structured exercises and is available as printed material or online and easily executed. The exercises consist of core stabilization, eccentric thigh muscle training, proprioceptive training, dynamic stabilization and plyometric exercises, all performed with proper postural alignment. The introduction of special exercises simulating escape manoeuvres, muscle strengthening and flexibility regarding the groin anatomic region could specifically complete this prevention programme.

5.7 Summary

Bullfighting is a controversial art that involves the man and the bull. Whenever people agree, or disagree, with this performing art, the reality is that it exists as a mixed of art performance and sports skills. Rigorous technical skills and optimal physical condition are the keys to minimize injuries that could be very serious and even mortal. Although there exists unpredictable specific injuries, namely, vascular serious lesions, most of the injuries could be trained through prevention programmes that should adopted by bullfighters.

References

1. Fiske-Harrison A. Perhaps bullfighting is not a moral wrong: My talk at the Edinburgh International Book Festival. In: The last arena: in search of the Spanish bullfight blog; 2012.
2. Hudson S. Sport and adventure tourism. Haworth Hospitality Press; 2003.
3. Rudloff U, Gonzalez V, Fernandez E, Holguin E, Rubio G, Lomelin J, Barrera R. Chirurgica Taurina: a 10-year experience of bullfight injuries. J Trauma Acute Care Surg. 2006;61(4):970–4.

Breakdance

6

Pauline Nouguès, Flora Petrot, and Patricia Thoreux

6.1 Introduction

Breakdance, also known as "breaking," is a street dance style, part of hip-Hop culture, which has emerged among African American and Puerto Rican populations in the 1970s in New York City, particularly in the Bronx [1].

At that time, the social climate of poverty and cultural diversity allowed the origin of the hip-hop movement and its various disciplines. This art consists of four elements: breaking, the dance element; MC, the vocal element (MC means "master of ceremonies" and is the one who raps/sings and hosts parties); graffiti, the art element; and DJ'ing, the music element (the DJ is responsible for producing and mixing the beats) [2].

Breakdance experienced a period of rapid growth in the 1980s with the beginning of the organization of international competitions known as "battles," which have contributed to the popularization of the discipline [1].

Today, it is considered as a fully-fledged art form and is practiced by thousands of people around the world. According to literature, more than 1 million people in the world practice breakdance, with approximately 11 international breakdance events and 560 national breakdance events each year [3]. In France, breakdance is included in the Dance Federation, and it is necessary to have a license to participate to any event.

In China, breakdance is a type of street dance. In 2013, the China Hip Hop Union Committee (CHUC) was founded by the Chinese Dancers Association, which allowed this art form to be recognized by the professional dance system and gained government support. It involves acrobatic and athletic movements performed to the rhythm of hip-hop music.

A dancer who is practicing breakdance is called a breakdancer, bboy or b-boy (for a man) bgirl or b-girl (for a woman), and it can be practiced in solo or as a team.

6.2 Specificities of Sport/Art

6.2.1 Techniques

Techniques are constantly evolving and, to a layman's eyes, are becoming more and more acrobatic. Dancers perform sequences when they dance. It begins with the toprock, a standing dance preparation step, followed by footwork or

P. Nouguès (✉)
INSEP, Paris 12th, Paris, France
e-mail: Pauline.NOUGUES@insep.fr

F. Petrot
INSEP/Department of Exercise and Sports Medicine, Jean Verdier Hospital, Bondy, France

P. Thoreux
Faculty of Health, UFR of Medicine, Université Paris Cité, Paris, France

CIMS (Center for Investigations in Sports Medicine), APHP, Hôtel Dieu Hospital, Paris, France

H. Jones, A. Lukaszenko (eds.), *Injury Prevention and Care in Artistic Sports*,
https://doi.org/10.1007/978-3-032-18105-3_6

downrock, a dance step performed on the ground where the dancer varies his or her footwork.

Some technical movements like drops, freezes and phases should be described as:

- *Drops* are transitional moves between toprock and footwork. Among the most common drops are:
  - The knee drop: from a standing position, the right leg lifts in hyperflexion, hooks behind the opposite knee, and lands on the ground in front of the knee.
  - The sweep drop or coin drop.
- *Freeze* is a static position that involves maintaining balance in an unstable position often supported on the upper limb or head (Figs. 6.1 and 6.2).
- *Phases* or power moves are the most acrobatic and aerial figures but can also be the most traumatic. They rely on repetitive circular movements of the legs, supported by the upper body (wrist, elbow, shoulder, head) where the dancer uses leg whips to initiate the rotation. They require a high level of personal skill and experience and often involve impacts with the ground.

"The Thomas" comes from gymnastics (pommel horse) and is used in breakdance on the ground: it is a circular movement using leg whips to create rotational force supported by axial compression on the wrists in hyperflexion and ulnar inclination (Fig. 6.3).

"The Crown" is a figure that uses the contour of the skull as a supporting surface. It involves a rotation made around the head initiated by the impulse of the upper body and accompanied by leg whips (Fig. 6.4).

"The Flare" is a figure where the dancer leans on one hand hyperextending the back performing circles with the legs while rotating the body (Fig. 6.5).

"The Headspin" is a figure where the dancer completes a full rotation on his head (Fig. 6.6).

6.2.2 Competition Runs

Athletes compete against each other by gender in one-to-one battles, combining physical and artistic performance. The dancers must adapt their

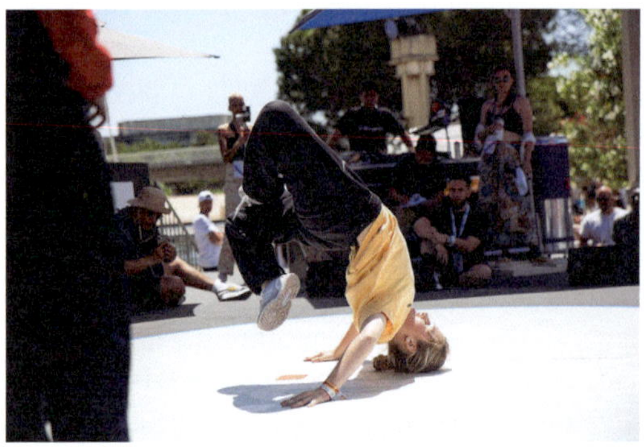

Fig. 6.2 Freeze by Bgirl Kimie @ Nassir Mokhtari—FFDanse. (Reproduced with permission)

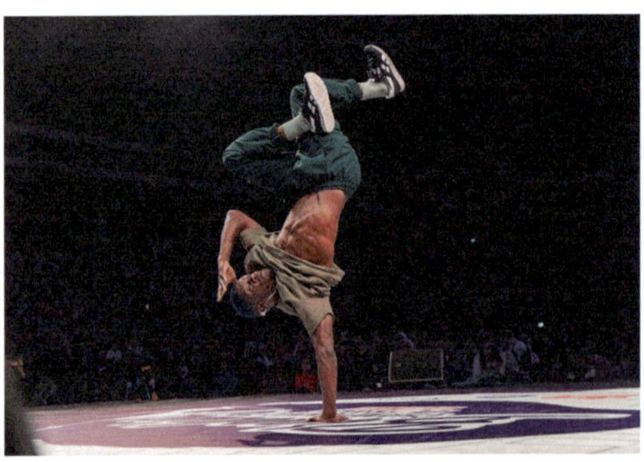

Fig. 6.1 Freeze by Bboy Dany Dan @ Nassir Mokhtari—FFDanse. (Reproduced with permission)

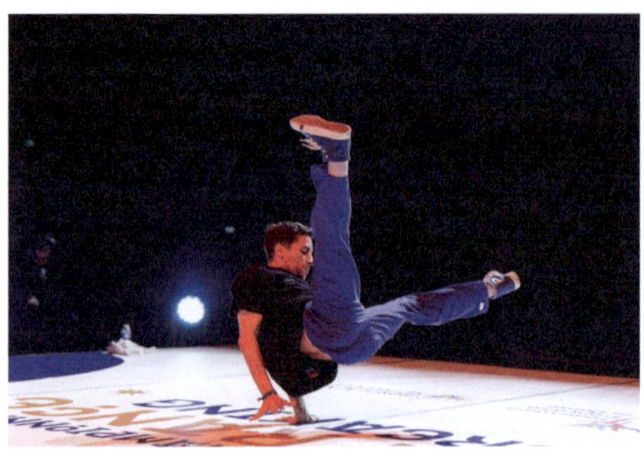

Fig. 6.3 The Thomas by Bboy Doudou @ Nassir Mokhtari—FFDanse. (Reproduced with permission)

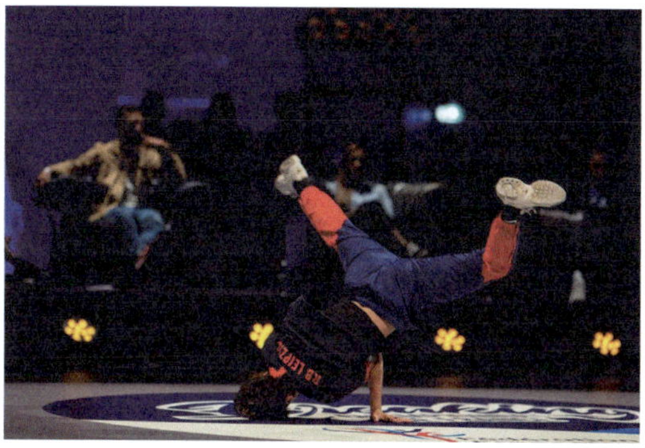

Fig. 6.4 The Crown by Bgirl Maessane @ Nassir Mokhtari—FFDanse. (Reproduced with permission)

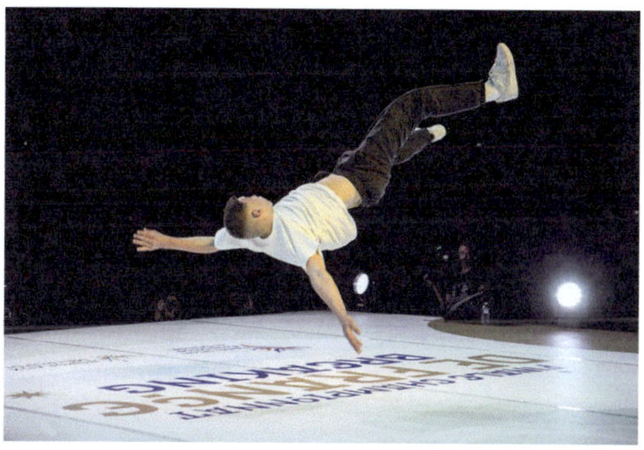

Fig. 6.5 The Flare by Bboy Marlone @ Nassir Mokhtari—FFDanse. (Reproduced with permission)

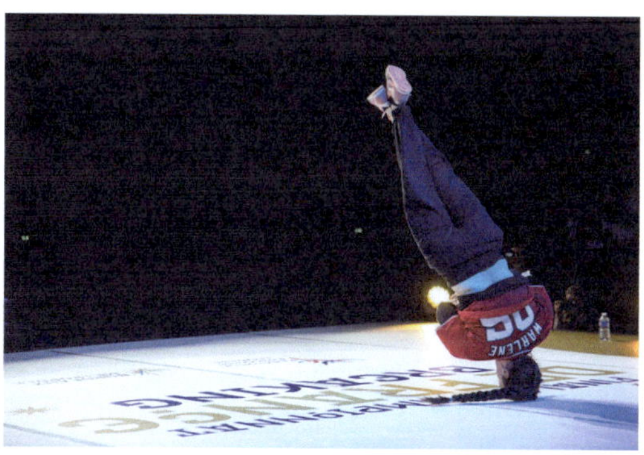

Fig. 6.6 The Headspin by Bgirl Warlene @ Nassir Mokhtari—FFDanse. (Reproduced with permission)

moves and improvise based on the DJ's music, which they are not familiar with in advance. Each dancer performs two rounds. A master of ceremonies organizes the proceedings of the competitions. One of his responsibilities is to enforce a 2-min break between each battle to allow the jury enough time to reach their verdict. The jury consists of three to five judges, always an odd number to minimize the possibility of ties. Specific points are not assigned to individual moves. The performance is analyzed based on four categories: attitude, top rock, footwork, and power moves.

At the end of the performances, the voting is done by a show of hands or digital responses depending on competition location. Each judge has a vote for "for" or "tie." In case of a tie, an additional round is performed to determine the winner. At this point, the "tie" vote is not allowed.

A part of the competition is called round-robin, which is a concept in which every participant dances against everyone. In a group round-robin, the participants are getting divided into different groups in which each participant battles each participant.

The big advantage of a group round-robin instead of direct knockout is that each participant has more opponents and therefore more chances to score more rounds and votes.

These rounds and votes are then used to create a round-robin ranking, ordered by the summary of rounds and the summary of votes. This provides a clear picture within every group.

A group of max four participants, resulting in six battles each group, is the best solution for breaking.

6.2.3 International Competitions

Several major international competitions have been organized each year since the 1990s.

Each competition takes the form of a contest, the outcome of which is voted on by a jury who selects the winner based on several criteria (musicality, technical performance, originality).

The BOTY (Battle Of The Year) is the flagship team competition held in Germany every year. The Red bull BC One, a solo competition, takes place in a different country each year.

Breakdancing was included in the program of the 2018 Youth Olympic Games in Buenos Aires and made its first official appearance on August

9–10, 2024, for the 2024 Olympic Games in Paris, in the emblematic Place de la Concorde in the center of Paris.

In 2020, French breakdancing joined the French Dance Federation, allowing breakdancers to obtain the status of high-level athletes in a view of the integration of this discipline into the Olympic Games. The French breakdance team has been based at the National Institute of Sport and Expertise since September 2022.

There were three qualifying competitions for those athletes seeking to compete in the 2024 Olympics Games:

The WDSF World Championship, which took place in Belgium in September 2023, with a quota of six places (three per gender) to award.

The Continental Games (Africa, Asia, Europe, Oceania, Pan-American) with a quota of ten places (five per gender) to award.

The Olympic Qualification Series (OQS), which took place from March to June 2024 and awarded the last 14 quota places available. As host country, France received two places.

At the Paris 2024 Olympics, the competition consisted of two events, one for men and one for women, with 16 B-Boys and 16 B-Girls competing for the first-ever Olympic-breaking title [4]. Each country could select at max two athletes per gender. France, as the host country, had at least two athletes (one per gender) automatically qualified.

6.3 Epidemiology of More Frequent Injuries

As in any sport, we find both joint and muscle injuries affecting the athlete's head, spine, upper limbs (shoulders, elbows, wrists, and fingers), and lower limbs (hips, knees, and ankles).

A recent study classified the main injury locations, and the following information emerged: wrist (20.31%, N = 26), ankle (15.63%, N = 20), knee (12.50%, N = 16), shoulder (10.94%, N = 14), and cervical spine (10.16%, N = 13). But there is limited epidemiological research available regarding this discipline. However, it has been shown that breakdance is more prone to injury than other dance styles. One study reported an injury rate of 4.02 injuries per 1000 h, with no significant difference between men and women. This discipline involves many complex acrobatic movements, which generate a great risk of injuries [5–9].

Neck pain is common and can be related to certain acrobatic figures such as headpins or falls.

Low-back pain is also a common complaint of breakdancers. The combination of footwork and fluid upper-body movements requires an increased demand on the trunk muscles. Imbalance in the core muscles is thought to be the cause of low-back pain, resulting in inappropriate muscle activation during repetitive, high-impact activities, such as those that occur throughout the breakdancing performance. Some breakdancing movements also require hyperextension of the back, such as "bridge" movements, resulting in an overload of the posterior joints. Concussions due to poor landing or headpin-type movements can also occur [10].

As the most mobile joint in the human body, the shoulder joint is very susceptible to injury due to its hyperlaxity and frequent instability. This discipline places repeated stress on this joint during choreography with rotations of the supporting hands in the closed kinetic chain movements of the dance. Chronic pain is frequently observed related to sub-acromial impingement with cuff tendinopathy, sub-acromioclavicular bursitis, or acromioclavicular arthritis.

In the elbows and wrists, we also find ligament and tendon damage [5–9].

Concerning hand injury, we are regularly confronted with phlyctens, dermabrasions, or even contusion due to impact and repeated support for rotational movements with figures such as spins or handstands.

Breakdance is a sport that includes fast and complex footwork, squats in forced hyper flexion, and knee twists with rapid changes of direction, mostly in unnatural body positions. An important part of the choreography also consists of acrobatic elements, where the dancers collide with the floor. All of these move-

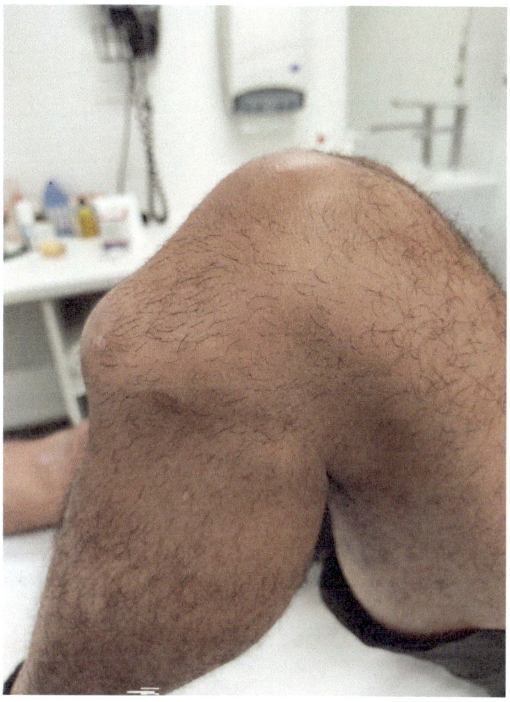

Fig. 6.7 Superficial prepatellar bursitis

ments present a high risk of knee injuries for these dancers. Among them, we frequently find ligament damage with sprains of the MCL and ACL, meniscal lesions, pre-patellar bursitis (Fig. 6.7) related to the supports, and dermabrasions. We can also find muscular lesions, such as in the adductor muscles.

6.4 Diagnosis

Making a diagnosis is not different from any other sport. It is mainly made by a clinical exam in correlation with the injured area. Based on this clinical assessment, appropriate additional examinations may be requested (X-rays, ultrasound, scanner, MRI, etc.) (Figs. 6.8, 6.9, 6.10, 6.11, and 6.12).

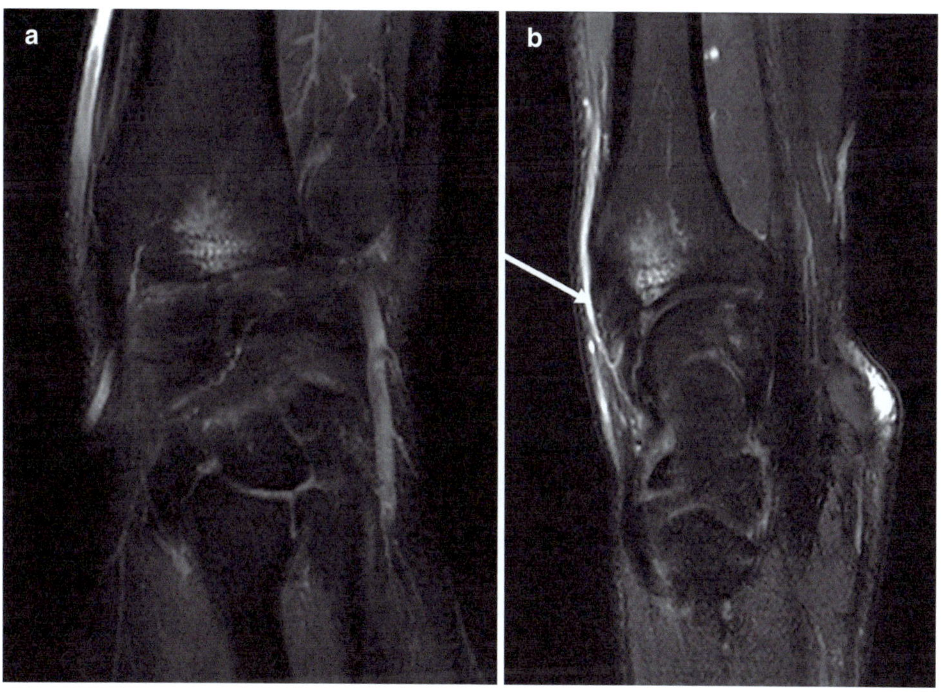

Fig. 6.8 MRI of a left wrist, coronal (**a**) and sagittal (**b**) proton density-weighted sequences with fat suppression: area of bone bruise with high signal intensity at the distal end of the radius on its dorsal side, associated with chronic extrinsic dorsal capsuloligamentous thickening of the radiocarpal joint (arrow), indicative of dorsal wrist impingement syndrome. (© INSEP Medical Imaging Department and its practitioners. Reproduced with permission)

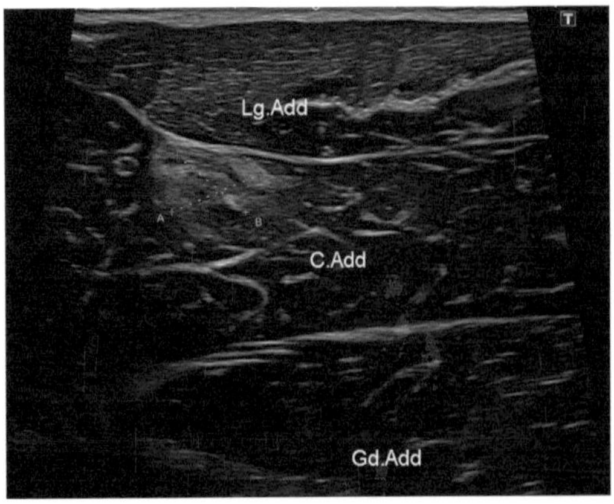

Fig. 6.9 Ultrasound of the right thigh: poorly defined hyperechoic area within the left adductor brevis muscle without disruption of muscle architecture, suggestive of a recent grade 1 M intrinsic lesion. (© INSEP Medical Imaging Department and its practitioners. Reproduced with permission)

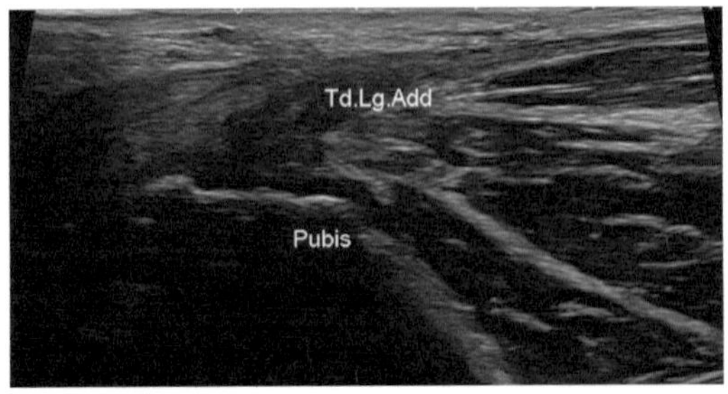

Fig. 6.10 Pubic ultrasound: thickening and deep hypoechoic focus of the left adductor longus tendon adjacent the pubic attachment, consistent with enthesopathy. (© INSEP Medical Imaging Department and its practitioners. Reproduced with permission)

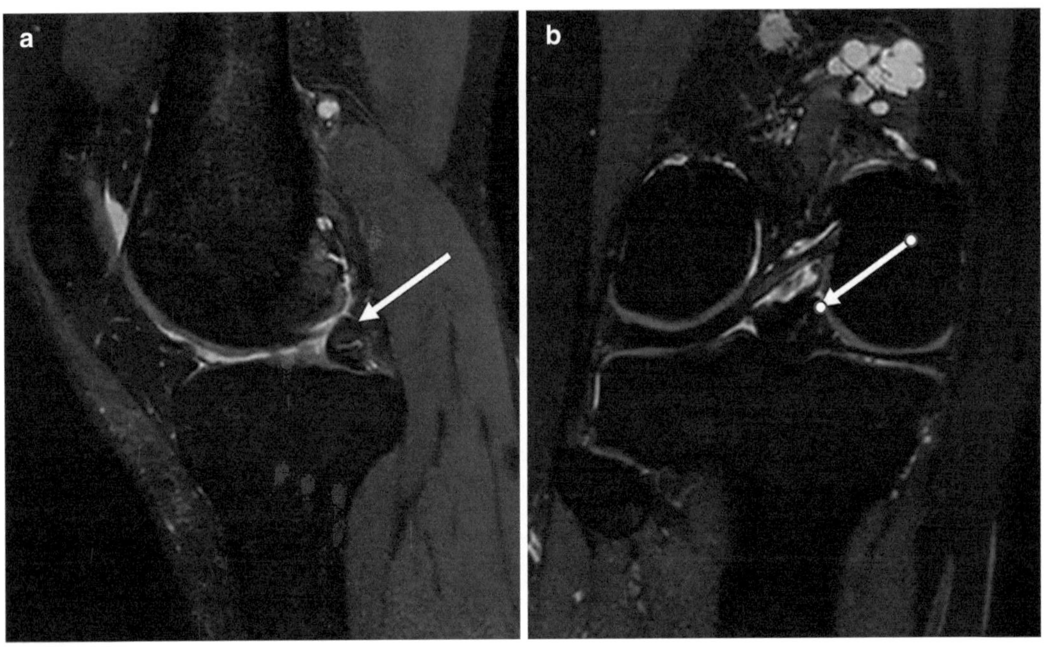

Fig. 6.11 MRI of a right knee, sagittal (**a**) and coronal (**b**) proton density-weighted sequences with fat suppression: medial meniscus tear with a large displaced meniscus in the notch (arrows). (© INSEP Medical Imaging Department and its practitioners. Reproduced with permission)

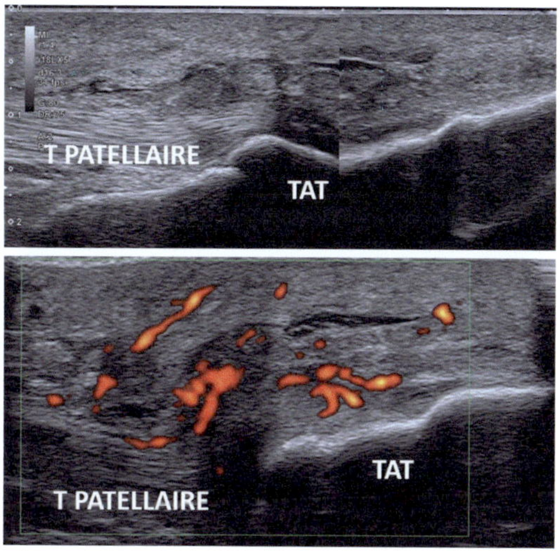

Fig. 6.12 Ultrasound of a right knee: marked hypoechoic thickening of the subcutaneous soft tissues adjacent to the distal attachment of the patellar tendon, with a thin fluid collection and significant vascularity on Doppler examination, consistent with bursitis. *TAT* anterior tibial tuberosity. (© INSEP Medical Imaging Department and its practitioners. Reproduced with permission)

6.5 Treatment Options

The treatment of breakdance injuries depends on their nature as well as their severity. The first step in treating an injury is to adjust the athletic load on the affected joint or even to rest it.

Icing an injury can help reduce inflammation of a joint. Sometimes, it is necessary to consider immobilization or compression of the injured area.

The administration of appropriate pain medication may also be prescribed (according to the anti-doping rules). Depending on the specific situations, physiotherapy will often be used depending on the specific situations [8].

6.6 RTP (Return to Performance)

Return to performance (RTP) corresponds to a key process involving returning an injured breakdance athlete to competition.

Depending on the injuries, a step-by-step rehabilitation protocol with a progression of return to dance must be defined. The emphasis is particularly placed on specific movement exercises for dancers and on objective clinical measures, in order to guide the progression of the return to dance.

6.7 Prevention

6.7.1 Injury Prevention

- Warm-up.
- Implementation of collective prevention measures.
  - Dynamic trunk control work.
  - Dynamic control of the pelvis with strengthening of lateral stabilizers of the pelvis and anti-valgus muscles.
  - Strengthening of the dorso-lumbar spine.
  - Core stability work with strengthening of deep abdominal muscles.
- Lower limb work.
  - Hip mobility.
  - Strengthening of IJ, adductor, and quadriceps.
  - Ankle mobility.
  - Strengthening of the sural triceps.
  - Intrinsic foot strengthening, inverters, everters.
- Upper limb work.
  - Strengthening of scapula stabilizers muscles.
  - Strengthening of rotator cuff muscle.
  - Shoulder mobility work.

In addition to these collective prevention groups, an individualized prevention program can be set up [8]:

Use of wrist, knee, and head protection: compression bandages or sleeves to reduce.

pressure and friction during movement,

Rest and recovery to improve performance and reduce the risk of injury.

Medical supervision by a medical staff composed of physiotherapists and sports doctors to help them adopt healthy practices.

6.7.2 Doping Prevention

Preventive measures can be put in place with athletes to combat doping:

- Awareness: it is vital to make athletes aware of the dangers of doping and the consequences it can have on their health and careers.
- Education: concerning different doping substances and methods.
- Doping controls: athletes must be informed that they may be subject to regular, random, and unannounced doping controls.

Every athlete is responsible for the substances detected in his or her urine or blood samples. A violation of the rules can be found even if the athlete has not acted intentionally.

It is the responsibility of the athletes and those around them to know what constitutes a rule violation. The World Anti-Doping Code (Articles 2.1 to 2.10), incorporated into the French Sports Code (Articles L. 232-9), specifies 11 types of anti-doping rule violation [11].

Anti-doping rule violations are not necessarily established just by the analysis of a sample taken during a doping control. For example, an athlete subject to mandatory whereabouts testing (target group) who misses three anti-doping tests within a 12-month period risks a suspension of 2 years [11].

References

1. Yang Z, Bai Y, Wei M. The importance of creativity in the sportification of breakdance. Front Educ. 2022;7:855724.
2. Ahassi C. Breakdance: del performance urbano al agenciamiento corporal. Tesis (Maestría en Estudios de la Cultura. Mención en Comunicación). Universidad Andina Simón Bolívar, Sede Ecuador. Área de Letras. 2009;94
3. Shapiro R. The aesthetics of institutionalization: breakdancing in France. J Arts Manag Law Soc. 2004;33:316–35.
4. Fédération Française de Danse. Chemin de sélection Breaking-Ranking/Paris2024? [En ligne]. Cited May 20, 2023. Available from: https://breaking.ffdanse.fr/comment-fonctionne-le-ranking-national/
5. Cho C, Song K, Min B, Lee S, et al. Musculoskeletal injuries in break-dancers. Injury. 2009;40(11):1207.
6. Joka T, Clarke N, Cohen D, al. Etiology of musculoskeletal injuries in amateur breakdancers. J Sports Med Phys Fitness. 2015;55(2):11.
7. Cousin F. Les Blessures liées à la pratique du Breakdance: étude épidémiologique transversale descriptive chez les danseurs amateurs et professionnels de plus de dix-huit ans. Thèse de médecine. Université de Caen, France; 2019.
8. Kauther M, Wedemeyer C, Wegner A, et al. Breakdance injuries and overuse syndromes in amateurs and professionals. Am J Sports Med. 2009;37(4):797–802.
9. Norman RA, Grodin MA. Injuries from break dancing. Am Fam Physician. 1984;30(4):109–12.
10. Stein CJ, Kinney SA, McCrystal T, al. Dance-related concussion: a case series. J Dance Med Sci. 2014;18(2):53–61.
11. AMA. World anti-doping Code. 2021. [Internet]. Cited May 20, 2023. Available from: https://www.wada-ama.org/sites/default/files/resources/files/wada_antidoping_code_2021_french_v9.pdf

Artistic Swimming 7

José Gomes Pereira

7.1 Introduction

Artistic swimming is a sport that involves elements of swimming, gymnastics, and dance and consists of the performance of a motor routine that includes complex and dynamic underwater movements executed according to choreographed music.

Some consider it one of the most demanding sports activities in the Olympic program due to its degree of difficulty and physical demand [1–3].

Based on Mountjoy et al. [4] and Viana et al. [5], the components of a synchronized swimmer's training include aerobic and anaerobic fitness, strength, power, endurance, flexibility, sport-specific skill perfection, artistic expression, and performance skills [2, 3, 6].

The present chapter aims to explore and comprehend the relationship between the training and competition load in artistic swimming and the associated medical issues, including diagnosis, treatment, and prevention. Artistic swimming is governed by the international federation FINA [7]. It showcases a variety of motor qualities such as strength, endurance, and flexibility, and coordinated actions performed in a choreographed manner, resulting in a visually impactful performance.

Artistic swimming, previously known as synchronized swimming, originated in the early twentieth century, with the first recorded competition in Berlin in 1891 [8]. Over time, the sport has evolved significantly due to rule changes and technical requirements. It gained recognition as an Olympic sport in 1984, solidifying its position as both an artistic expression and a physically demanding athletic activity [2, 3, 6, 9].

The core foundation of artistic swimming lies in synchronized motor activities and harmonious collective coordination among team members. Beyond athleticism, artistic swimming conveys emotions and narratives through choreography.

Swimmers use facial expressions, body language, and gestures to express emotions and enhance performance. Using costumes, props, and makeup contributes to the sport's thematic and visually appealing nature. Artistic swimming is a sport and a remarkable form of artistic expression.

The physiological characterization of artistic swimming is important for the medical aspects of the sport for several reasons. Concerning injury prevention, it is essential to understand the physiological demands of artistic swimming to identify potential injury risks and the subsequent implementation of injury prevention strategies. By studying the physiological characteristics of

J. G. Pereira (✉)
Desporsano Sports Clinic, Lisbon, Portugal

H. Jones, A. Lukaszenko (eds.), *Injury Prevention and Care in Artistic Sports*,
https://doi.org/10.1007/978-3-032-18105-3_7

successful swimmers, medical professionals can help optimize training programs and individualize them for athletes. This includes tailoring strength and conditioning exercises, designing cardiovascular training plans, and monitoring performance markers.

The physiological demands of artistic swimming necessitate appropriate nutritional strategies to support energy expenditure, muscle recovery, and overall health [10, 11]. By understanding the metabolic requirements of the sport, medical professionals can provide targeted guidance on optimal nutrition and hydration strategies.

In injury management and rehabilitation, injuries can still occur in artistic swimming despite preventive measures. Understanding the physiological demands of the sport allows medical professionals to provide effective rehabilitation programs. They can also develop return-to-play protocols to ensure a safe and successful return to training and competition.

Monitoring Health and Well-Being: Regular physiological assessments can help monitor artistic swimmers' overall health and well-being. Medical professionals can identify signs of overtraining, fatigue, and other health issues by tracking physiological markers, such as heart rate variability, lactate levels, body composition, and hormonal profiles. The possibility of implementing early intervention reduces the risk of medical conditions contributing to and optimizing performance.

From a general medical and sports medicine perspective, artistic swimming places a high physiological demand on athletes, combining cardiopulmonary fitness and musculoskeletal activity elements. Consequently, medical issues can arise, ranging from functional problems to musculoskeletal injuries. Some authors have described the mental health benefits associated with artistic swimming. Given the complexity of the sport, its demands are substantial, often resulting in sport-specific injuries. Therefore, it is essential from a medical standpoint to understand the fundamental structure of artistic swimming and its requirements, as these factors can often explain the common injuries encountered [4]. This chapter aims to provide a physiological and medical characterization of artistic swimming.

7.2 Physiological Characterization of Artistic Swimming

Artistic swimming is a highly unique and demanding sport involving choreographed routines performed in water, with athletes executing various movements above and below the water surface (Fig. 7.1a, b).

According to several studies [2, 7, 12], evidence supports the notion that elite athletes in artistic swimming possess certain advantages related to their respiratory systems. One of the findings suggests that elite athletes have an increased resistance to hypoxia (low oxygen levels). This implies that these athletes have a greater

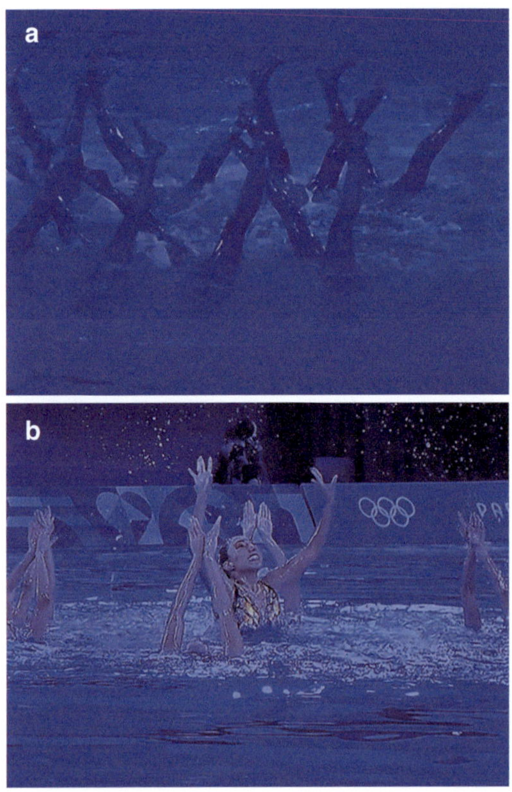

Fig. 7.1 Movements above water (**a**) and below water (**b**)

capacity to endure and adapt to situations where oxygen levels may be lower, which can be beneficial during the physically demanding routines of artistic swimming. Additionally, Rovnaya et al. [13] discovered a positive relationship between the functionality of the external respiratory system and performance level in artistic swimming. As the respiratory system's functionality improves, an athlete's performance in artistic swimming also tends to increase.

One of the critical aspects of artistic swimming with significant physiological impact is the extended periods of breath-holding underwater.

7.3 Physiologic Consequences of Breath-Holding

Breath-holding and underwater activity produce several acute and chronic adaptations. It creates a physiological environment where gas exchange is limited, resulting in reduced oxygen availability and increased carbon dioxide accumulation, with implications for the respiratory, cardiovascular, and neurological systems.

During breath-holding, the accumulation of CO_2 due to the inability to expel it can reduce pH levels in the blood and muscle tissue, impairing performance [14]. The respiratory system may change to adapt to the increased demands of breath-holding; furthermore, the number and duration of underwater exposures can influence the perceived exertion difficulty [15]. The physiological adaptations and the associated challenges faced by athletes in this sport require careful training and preparation and an understanding of the body's responses to breath-holding.

Athletes must perform complex and strenuous movements while breathing, significantly demanding their cardiovascular and respiratory systems [7, 11, 12]. This leads to a physiological adaptation known as the bradycardic response. The bradycardic response is characterized by a decrease in heart rate during prolonged breath-holding. This response is an adaptive mechanism that helps conserve oxygen and maintain physiological function while the athlete is underwater [7, 11, 12] (Fig. 7.2).

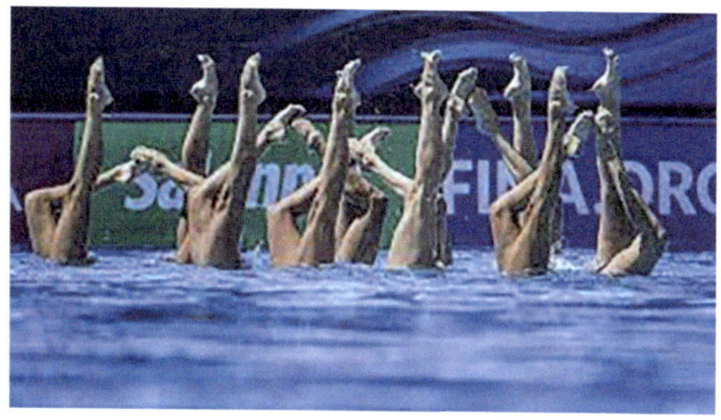

Fig. 7.2 Underwater adaptation breath control

The body's natural response to breath-holding is to slow down the heart rate, which reduces oxygen consumption and allows the athlete to stay underwater for longer durations. This truly influences training prescription and desired training outcomes [5].

In artistic swimming, some key aspects lie in cardiorespiratory fitness, which plays a vital role in training and performance. As artistic swimming involves continuous movement and the execution of apnea routines, swimmers must have high aerobic capacity and power [16]. They perform intricate routines underwater while holding their breath for extended periods. This prolonged breath-hold can have several physiological consequences for the body [17]. The longer the breath-hold is, the lower the oxygen levels become, which can impact overall performance and limit the duration of the routine.

If the breath-holding continues, carbon dioxide levels in the body increase. Hypercapnia can lead to discomfort and a breathing urge, ultimately triggering the body's natural response to breathing [18].

Prolonged breath-holding leads to various physiological changes, including bradycardia (a decrease in heart rate), peripheral vasoconstriction, and redistribution of blood to the brain and heart.

It is important to note that breath-holding, especially in the context of underwater activities, can lead to several physiological consequences and adaptations [17, 18]. These effects primarily arise from the limitation of gas exchange. During breath-hold, the ability to exchange gases (oxygen and carbon dioxide) is reduced. The combination of limited gas exchange and intense muscle contractions places additional physiological stress on the body [19].

As breath-holding continues, carbon dioxide accumulates in the blood and muscle tissue [20]. This leads to a rise in the partial pressure of carbon dioxide (pCO_2). The accumulation of CO_2 contributes to decreased pH levels (acidosis).

The reduction in oxygen availability is related to a decreased tendency of the partial pressure of oxygen (pO_2), impacting cognitive function and decision-making [21, 22]. In this case, the performer may experience dulled consciousness, which has an impact on the performance, increasing the number of errors in the technical performance [22].

With decreased oxygen supply, holding the breath underwater does not permit replenishing the oxygen supply. The tendency to lower your body's oxygen levels grows more pronounced the longer you hold your breath. This can lead to oxygen deprivation or hypoxia [23, 24].

Blood redistribution also suffers alterations: When you submerge in water, your body initiates a series of physiological responses known as the diving reflex. This underwater reflex can cause blood vessels in the extremities to constrict, redirecting blood flow to vital organs like the heart and brain. This mechanism helps conserve oxygen and enables longer breath-holding times. However, it can also reduce circulation to the limbs and extremities.

In chronotropic adaptation and blood pressure, the heart rate and blood pressure may gradually rise as the longer breath-holding continues, conditioning additional impact on the cardiovascular system.

The baroreceptor activity in the major blood vessels responds to changes in blood pressure. When you hold your breath, the baroreceptors detect the increase in pressure caused by the cardiovascular response. This can trigger reflexes to lower blood pressure, such as vasodilation and a decrease in heart rate. These reflexes can also contribute to the redistribution of blood flow [24, 25].

These respiratory adaptations to repeated apnea can allow athletes competing in artistic swimming to hold their breath longer and at a lower HR despite experiencing more significant reductions in SaO_2 and similar changes in alveolar gases as controls [17]. The respiratory adaptations in artistic swimmers, when compared to controls, have been documented [9, 10]; however, the relationship between cardio-respiratory parameters such as forced vital capacity (FVC) and FEV1, and performance level suggests further investigation [13].

Although specific data on blood lactate and oxygen consumption values in artistic swimming are limited, some general assumptions can be made considering the physiological demands.

What are the long-term physiological consequences of practicing artistic swimming? How can athletes train to improve their respiratory systems? What are the potential risks associated with prolonged breath-holding in artistic swimming?

Concerning blood lactate [3], artistic swimming involves intense aerobic and anaerobic activities, including sustained swimming with the production of lactic acid and lactate in the muscles. At the same time, lactate values can vary depending on the individual athlete and the intensity of training or performance. Blood lactate levels can rise significantly during intense training, and values above 8–10 mmol/L have been reported in some studies. This suggests a high anaerobic component and indicates that the athletes perform at or near their maximum capacity. During moderate training, blood lactate levels might range between 2 and 6 mmol/L, indicating a mix of aerobic and anaerobic metabolism [3].

Oxygen consumption (VO2) measures the volume of oxygen an individual consumes per minute during exercise and indicates aerobic fitness and energy expenditure. While there is limited research on artistic swimming, we can draw upon studies on swimming and similar aquatic activities. Oxygen consumption can be high, ranging from 40 to 60 ml/kg/min. These values indicate a high aerobic demand and the athletes' ability to utilize oxygen efficiently. During moderate training or routines, oxygen consumption might range between 20 and 40 ml/kg/min, depending on the intensity and duration of the activity. These values can vary based on individual fitness, training status, and the specific demands of the routine or training session. The above values are general estimations, and actual measurements may vary among individuals [19].

Davis et al. [26] and Jamnik et al. [27] demonstrated that artistic swimmers are exposed to considerable metabolic demand because of the combination of BH and vigorous exercise. Results from Rodríguez-Zamora et al. [3] indicated moderate-to-high La peak in junior and senior-age categories, ranging from 5 to 13 mmol·L $^{-1}$, with an overall average of 7.3 mmol·L $^{-1}$ as the mean across all routines. This possibly indicates a considerable anaerobic contribution to the sport. Interestingly, Jamnik et al. [27] reported an average La of 12.7 ± 1.3 mmol·L $^{-1}$. This finding might indicate that high-level performers can better tolerate increases in metabolic acidosis or represent a greater glycolytic demand [21].

Concerning apnea and anaerobic performances, artistic swimming often involves periods of breath-holding or reduced breathing. This requires anaerobic energy production, as the body relies on stored energy sources, such as creatine phosphate and glycogen, to meet the demands of intense movements without a sufficient oxygen supply. The available literature has estimated the anaerobic contributions through excess post-exercise oxygen consumption (EPOC) during the first 3 min of recovery. Bante et al. [28] speculated that the EPOC was used for phosphocreatine synthesis. Consequently, prolonged and repeated apneic exposures may increase the anaerobic contributions of Rodríguez and Mader [29].

7.4 The Bradycardic Response

The bradycardic response associated with breath-holding in water is the mammalian dive reflex. It represents a set of physiological changes that occur in humans when they submerge. The first significant change during breath-holding is the trigeminal nerve activation, which is responsible for facial sensations. The brainstem triggers the parasympathetic nervous system. This activation leads to a decrease in heart rate, known as bradycardia. The purpose of this response is to conserve oxygen and redirect blood flow to vital organs, such as the heart and brain, during submersion [30].

The bradycardic response is often more pronounced in trained divers or individuals who regularly engage in breath-holding activities. These individuals may experience a more significant reduction in heart rate and a more efficient blood flow distribution during breath-holding in water.

It is important to note that the mammalian dive reflex is a complex physiological response that involves multiple factors. The exact mechanisms and extent of the bradycardic response can vary between individuals [31].

One significant challenge is the bradycardic response triggered by prolonged periods of breath-holding. Athletes must hold their breath while engaging in physically demanding activities in this discipline [19]. The combination of breath-holding and submersion in water has various implications for gas exchange, particularly when coupled with intense muscular activity. Consequently, a physiological environment characterized by compromised gas exchange emerges due to extended apnea periods, resulting in hypercapnia and reduced oxygen availability [12, 13]. Under normal physiological conditions, respiration is regulated by chemoreceptors that respond to elevated CO_2 levels [13]. Conversely, a decrease in pH is associated with hypercapnia since CO_2 cannot be expelled through expiration, leading to lactic acidosis and hypoxic training. This situation can hinder performance by impacting cognitive function, decision-making, and consciousness, affecting sports performance [30].

7.5 The Aerobic Capacity

Aerobic capacity refers to the ability of the cardiovascular system to transport and deliver oxygen to the working muscles during exercise. By improving aerobic capacity, swimmers can enhance their endurance and sustain high-intensity performances for extended periods. This is important for artistic swimmers, as they engage in routines that require continuous movement, such as synchronized swimming routines.

In addition to continuous movement, artistic swimmers perform routines involving breath-holding or apnea. These routines require efficient oxygen utilization and the ability to withstand breath-holding periods. Developing a robust cardiovascular system is crucial for supplying oxygen to the working muscles during apnea routines and removing metabolic by-products that can accumulate during these periods.

Training for anaerobic performance involves high-intensity interval training, sprinting, and specific breath-holding exercises. Programs for artistic swimmers typically focus on improving aerobic endurance. These programs often involve activities such as interval training and endurance-based exercises. Swimmers may also engage in activities like running or cycling to enhance their aerobic capacity.

A high maximal oxygen uptake (VO2 max) is essential for aerobic capacity. Most studies conducted on artistic swimmers have focused on examining VO2 max. Roby et al. [10] reported an average VO2 max of 43 ml/kg/min and concluded that aerobic capacity did not play a crucial role in artistic swimming performance. Furthermore, it has been suggested that artistic swimming necessitates both aerobic and anaerobic power, primarily due to the lengthy apneic periods spent underwater during strenuous movements [9, 23]. Anaerobic capacity is typically determined through maximal exercise tests. The lack of a significant correlation between anaerobic capacity and performance scores may stem from the low specificity of conventional anaerobic tests.

By consistently working on their cardiorespiratory fitness, artistic swimmers can improve their overall performance, enhance their endurance, and meet the physical demands of their sport more effectively.

To improve aerobic capacity, training programs often incorporate the principles of progressive overload and specificity. Progressive overload involves gradually increasing the intensity, duration, or frequency of aerobic exercise to challenge the cardiovascular and respiratory systems. Factors like age, genetics, body composition, and prior training history also impact aerobic capacity. While genetics play a role, most individuals can improve their aerobic capacity through regular exercise. Periodization is a strategy commonly used in training programs to optimize performance gains.

Within aerobic performance and exercises conducted with oxygen deficiency, training in hypoxia helps swimmers develop breathing control techniques that enable them to stay underwater for extended periods during their artistic swimming routines. Swimmers can maintain a rhythmic pattern by optimizing lung capacity and controlling breathing while executing complex movements. Over time, artistic swimming has become increasingly demanding, presenting unique challenges to athletes.

7.6 The Adaptive Training Process

David Bentley et al. [32], exploring the physiological response during an artistic swimming routine, confirmed the severity of underwater swimming and found that the movement rate significantly increased the metabolic demand of the routine. This information is crucial for designing effective training programs and determining the appropriate training load for artistic swimmers.

Based on the same author, understanding the metabolic demands of the routine can help athletes optimize their energy systems and improve their overall performance. The study suggests that further research is necessary to investigate the long-term changes in metabolic response and performance parameters.

Ponciano et al. [19] systematically reviewed the scientific literature on physiological responses in synchronized swimmers between 2006 and 2016 to analyze physiological responses in artistic swimmers, either during competitions or laboratory tests. The measurements included lactate levels, heart rate [31], rates of perceived exertion, VO2, and lung volume.

For these authors, the standardization of instruments and definitions is crucial for advancing scientific knowledge.

Artistic swimmers develop unique physiological adaptations during adaptive training due to repeated exposure to apnea-induced efforts [18]. These adaptations are reflected in enhanced pulmonary function and noticeable bradycardic response [32]. Artistic swimming also entail demanding metabolic adaptations, as indicated by peak blood lactate levels (La peak) reaching approximately 13 mmol·L $^{-1}$, with an average of 7.3 mmol·L $^{-1}$ overall. These values suggest a substantial anaerobic contribution. This anaerobic contribution is evident through excess post-exercise oxygen consumption (EPOC) during the initial 3 min of recovery, along with lactate measurements [3, 16].

Yamamura et al. [23] investigate the relationship between physiological characteristics and performance scores in artistic swimmers. The variables examined in the study included body dimensions, body composition, isokinetic muscle strength of the elbow and knee during extension and flexion, abdominal muscle endurance, anaerobic power (leg extension power and peak blood lactate concentration), aerobic power (maximum oxygen uptake [VO2max], swimming velocity at the onset of blood lactate accumulation [OBLA-V]), and flexibility (standing trunk flexion, prone trunk extension, and distance between the open legs).

Maintaining balance and proprioceptive activity is crucial for achieving spatiotemporal awareness while executing intricate artistic actions, such as inverted positions in water, often without direct visual reference points. In training programs, swimmers must also acclimate themselves to water temperatures and develop strategies to maintain homeostasis during prolonged periods in the water.

Various studies suggest that functional aspects such as muscle strength, endurance, and aerobic capacity are critical determinants of performance scores in artistic swimmers. This highlights the significance of physiological factors over anthropometric variables with performance. Yamamura et al. [23] suggest that functional aspects such as muscle strength, muscle endurance, and aerobic capacity are fundamental determinants of performance scores in artistic swimmers, highlighting the significance of physiological factors over anthropometric variables about performance [12, 26]. It is also essential to consider that artistic swimmers often use training techniques to improve their flexibility and overall performance (Fig. 7.3).

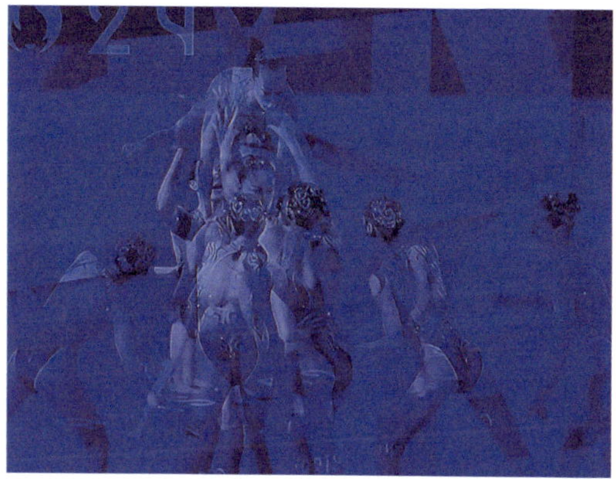

Fig. 7.3 Training techniques for coordination, flexibility, and performance are fundamental

Active stretching involves actively contracting muscles opposite those being stretched. Passive stretching involves external forces (e.g., a partner, gravity, or equipment) providing the stretching force. PNF techniques involve a combination of muscle contraction and relaxation to enhance flexibility. Yoga and Pilates can help improve core stability, body control, and flexibility through specific movements and poses.

Due to the physically demanding nature of artistic swimming, injury prevention is crucial [1, 4]. There are typical injuries of this modality that will be discussed further ahead.

7.7 Injuries and Medical Problems in Artistic Swimming

Artistic swimming is a physically demanding sport that offers exciting challenges for sports medicine specialists. It presents excellent research potential, considering the scarcity of published literature on the subject due to its specific characteristics, and creates conditions for the emergence of medical problems [1, 4, 6].

In artistic swimming, the mandatory technical elements illustrate the athlete's flexibility, strength, skill, power, and motor control. The training pattern is high volume and high intensity. The training program is designed to balance the following components: fitness building, acquiring sports-specific skills, normal development, routine perfection, and recovery. The skills required in artistic swimming include flexibility, aerobic and anaerobic endurance, core strength, power, acrobatics, strength, endurance, choreography skills, and artistic expression [33]. Under these training procedures and competitions, there are risk factors for common injuries that can occur in the practice of artistic swimming.

7.8 Type of Injuries, Treatment Management, and Return to Play

7.8.1 Acute

Artistic swimming was once thought of as a non-contact sport, where injuries were acquired from either outside the sport or from repetitive chronic overuse injuries. With the recent advances in the high risk of some technical performances, there has been an increase in the incidence of traumatic injuries. Serious head injuries with post-concussive syndrome have also been seen [34]. Acute tears of muscles and tendons occur with the increase in high-speed, ballistic movements. The two most common musculoskeletal overuse injuries encountered in clinical practice among elite artistic swimmers are shoulder instability problems and lumbar strains [33, 35].

The evolution and specific demands of training and competitions in artistic swimming require developing high-risk acrobatic skills, especially in team routines. Athletes often risk traumatic injuries through contact with another swimmer or on the pool deck.

Athletes train for these skills on dry land using mats, and injuries can occur during training if proper safety precautions are not followed. This new trend in synchronized swimming has resulted in a shift in acute injuries, including concussions, bruises, sprains/strains, herniated discs, and fractures [36, 37]. Acute muscle and tendon ruptures occur with increased high-speed ballistic movements. The team physician needs to be familiar with the latest guidelines for concussion treatment due to the high training load [5, 12].

The evolution and specific demands of training and competitions in artistic swimming require developing high-risk acrobatic skills, especially in team routines. Acute traumatic injuries are physical injuries that occur suddenly due to an external force or impact. These injuries can affect various body parts, including bones, muscles, ligaments, tendons, organs, and the central nervous system.

The fractures are relatively common and refer to broken or cracked bones. They frequently result from trauma or excessive force applied to the bone, such as falls, accidents, or sports injuries. Fractures can vary in severity, ranging from hairline cracks to complete breaks where the bone is separated into two or more pieces. The closed fractures show a broken bone, but the skin remains intact.

In an open fracture, the bone pierces through the skin, leading to an open wound. This type of fracture carries a higher risk of infection. In comminuted fracture, the bone breaks into multiple fragments. Hairline fracture involves a small crack in the bone that may not be easily visible on X-rays.

Stress fracture is a hairline crack that occurs due to repetitive stress or overuse of a particular bone. These fractures are often seen in athletes. The symptoms of a fracture can include pain, swelling, bruising, deformity, difficulty moving the affected area, and sometimes an audible sound or sensation at the time of injury. Diagnosis is typically made through physical examination, X-rays, and occasionally other imaging tests like MRI or CT scans. Treatment for fractures depends on the type and severity of the fracture. It can include immobilization with casts, splints, or braces to allow the bone to heal correctly. In some cases, surgical intervention can be necessary to realign the bone fragments or stabilize the fracture with implants like screws, plates, or rods. Rehabilitation, including physical therapy, may also be necessary to restore strength and mobility after the bone has healed.

Sprains happen when a ligament, which connects bone to bone, is stretched or torn. This injury often occurs in joints such as the ankles, wrists, or knees and can be caused by sudden twisting or overextension.

Strains occur when a muscle or tendon connecting muscle to bone is overstretched or torn. Sudden movements, excessive force, or repetitive activities can cause it. Common strains include hamstring strains and pulled muscles.

Contusions, also known as bruises, happen when blood vessels under the skin rupture due to a direct impact or trauma. They result in discoloration, swelling, and pain in the affected area.

Concussions are traumatic brain injuries affecting the head or severe body shaking. They can lead to temporary loss of consciousness, headaches, dizziness, confusion, and other neurological symptoms [14].

Dislocations occur when the bones forming a joint are forced out of their normal position. A strong impact or abnormal movement often causes this injury, resulting in severe pain, swelling, and immobility of the affected joint.

Penetrating injuries happen when an object pierces through the skin and damages underlying tissues, organs, or structures. These injuries require immediate medical attention due to the potential for internal bleeding and infection.

Medical attention is essential for acute traumatic injuries, especially if they are severe or involve the head, neck, spine, or major organs. Proper diagnosis, treatment, and rehabilitation are essential for recovery and to minimize long-term complications.

Athletes usually train for these skills on dry land using mats, and injuries can occur during training if proper safety precautions are not followed. This new trend in artistic swimming has resulted in a shift in acute injuries, including concussions, bruises, sprains/strains, herniated discs, and fractures [36, 37]. Acute muscle and tendon ruptures occur with increased high-speed ballistic movements. The team physician needs to be familiar with the latest guidelines for concussion treatment [34, 38] due to the high training load.

7.9 Overuse Injuries

Overuse injuries are due to repetitive stress on a particular part of the body without sufficient recovery time. These injuries are common among athletes and individuals who engage in repetitive activities or movements. Studies on overuse injuries in artistic swimming are scarce, but the injury is relatively standard. However, the prevalence of overuse injuries is not documented in the scientific literature. Four body regions are most commonly affected in artistic swimming: the shoulder, lumbar and cervical spine, and the knee [33, 35, 38, 39].

To prevent overuse injuries, it is important to incorporate proper training techniques, such as gradually increasing the intensity and duration of activities and taking rest days; it is also crucial to listen to your body and pay attention to warning signs of pain or discomfort. Treatment may include rest, physical therapy, pain management, and modifying activities for adequate recovery.

The diagnosis of overuse injuries typically involves a combination of medical history, physical examination, and sometimes imaging studies. Here are the critical steps involved in diagnosing overuse injuries:

Medical history: Exploring symptoms, the duration and pattern of pain or discomfort, and any activities or movements aggravating or alleviating the symptoms. They may also inquire about your exercise routine, training regimen, or any recent changes in activity levels.

A careful physical examination will look for inflammatory signs. They may palpate the area to identify tender points, assess the range of motion, and check for muscle imbalances or weakness.

Imaging studies: In some cases, imaging studies like X-rays, ultrasound, magnetic resonance imaging (MRI), or computed tomography (CT) scans may be ordered to visualize the affected area more closely. These imaging techniques can help identify stress fractures, ligament or tendon damage, or other structural abnormalities.

Differential diagnosis: Overuse injuries can have similar symptoms to other conditions, so it's important to rule out alternative diagnoses. The healthcare provider may consider conditions such as tendonitis, bursitis, stress fractures, muscle strains, nerve impingements, or arthritis.

Specialized tests: Depending on the suspected diagnosis, additional specialized tests may be performed. These could include electromyography (EMG) to assess nerve function, bone scans to detect stress fractures, or arthroscopy to examine joint structures in more detail.

Treatment typically involves a combination of rest, activity modification, physical therapy, pain management, and sometimes surgical intervention in severe cases.

7.10 Collisions and Concussions

Collisions between swimmers can happen due to miscommunication, crowded routines, or challenging lifts and throws. These collisions may result in severe damage [39].

Although not as common as other injuries on this list, concussions can occur in artistic swimming if swimmers hit their heads on the bottom of the pool or collide with other swimmers during lifts or other moves.

In artistic swimming, collisions can occasionally occur, although they are relatively rare. Nevertheless, given the intricate and precise movements involved in artistic swimming routines, collisions can happen when swimmers misjudge their positioning or timing. These collisions can occur between teammates or swimmers from different teams during competitions.

While collisions may disrupt the flow and synchronization of the routine, they are generally accidental. Swimmers train extensively to maintain spatial awareness and coordination to minimize the risk of collisions. However, due to the complex nature of the sport, occasional collisions can still happen.

When a collision occurs, the swimmers involved usually try to regain their composure and quickly adapt to the situation, often making adjustments on the spot to continue the routine as seamlessly as possible. To mitigate the risk of collisions, coaches and swimmers work together to create routines that minimize the chances of accidental contact. They also focus on improving communication and coordination among team members to ensure smooth transitions and synchronized movements.

It is essential to take care of the safety and conduct of swimmers during competitions. Officials closely monitor routines to ensure they adhere to the established guidelines and may penalize teams for collisions or any other violations that occur during a performance.

While collisions can occur in artistic swimming, they are infrequent and unintended. Swimmers and coaches prioritize safety, coordination, and precision to create visually stunning and synchronized routines.

While concussions are not as common in artistic swimming as in contact sports like football or rugby, they can still occur due to accidental collisions or falls during training or competition.

First of all, the recognition of the medical importance of the situation is important, but also education for athletes, coaches, and officials to recognize the signs and symptoms of a concussion. This includes understanding the potential risks and consequences of participating in the sport while being concussed [35].

Athletes should be encouraged to promptly report any suspected concussions to their coach or medical staff. The athlete should be immediately removed from training or competition and evaluated by a medical professional experienced in concussion management. Physical and cognitive rest are typically recommended initially to allow the brain to heal. A gradual return-to-play progression should be followed, ensuring the athlete is symptom-free before increasing activity levels.

Concerning the Return-to-Play Protocol, once the athlete is symptom-free and has completed the appropriate rest and recovery period, they can begin a gradual return-to-play protocol under the guidance of a healthcare professional. The return-to-play progression should involve increasing activity levels while monitoring for any recurrence of symptoms [35].

It is crucial to follow a step-by-step approach to minimize the risk of re-injury or complications. For specific guidelines and protocols related to artistic swimming and concussions, it is advisable to consult the governing bodies of the sport, such as the International Swimming Federation (FINA), and qualified medical professionals specializing in sports-related concussions.

7.11 Shoulder Problems

The activity of artistic swimming occurs repetitively for several hours daily. It is hard training. All of these repetitive actions over time may result in micro-trauma to the rotator cuff, particularly the supraspinatus, and sometimes to the long head of the biceps. Another mechanism may be the impingement of inflamed soft tissue structures, such as the subacromial bursa, within the anatomical constraints of the subacromial space. Treatment of this injury requires an understanding of the demands on the shoulder in synchronized swimming. To ensure adequate shoulder rest, the athlete must be limited from performing freestyle and other activities that place the shoulder in the vulnerable impingement position [40].

The shoulder joint is particularly vulnerable in artistic swimming due to the frequent overhead movements and lifts performed in routines. Swimmers can develop conditions such as shoulder impingement, rotator cuff injuries, or labral tears, mostly due to repetitive overhead movements and intense training in the sport. Diagnosing, treating, and preventing shoulder injuries in artistic swimmers require a multifaceted approach. However, a healthcare professional must give medical advice and look for an accurate diagnosis and personalized treatment plan [40].

For the diagnosis and physical examination, the healthcare provider will assess the shoulder, looking for signs of inflammation, swelling, instability, or limited range of motion. They may also test muscle strength and perform special tests to evaluate specific structures in the shoulder joint.

Imaging tests: X-rays, magnetic resonance imaging (MRI), or ultrasound may be ordered to visualize the internal structures of the shoulder and rule out other potential causes of pain or injury.

For the treatment, rest and activity modification are recommended; reducing or modifying activities exacerbating shoulder pain is crucial for healing. It may involve temporary cessation of artistic swimming or modification of training routines.

Physical therapy: Should be designed a rehabilitation program tailored to your injury. It may include exercises to strengthen the rotator cuff muscles, improve shoulder stability, and enhance flexibility.

Medications: Nonsteroidal anti-inflammatory drugs (NSAIDs) or analgesics may reduce pain and inflammation.

Injection therapy: In some cases, platelet-rich plasma (PRP) injections may be used to alleviate pain and promote healing.

Surgical intervention: Severe cases of a shoulder injury, for example, a rotator cuff tear or labral tear, may require surgical repair.

Prevention: Proper technique and training: Ensure you use the correct technique during movements and lifts to minimize excessive stress on the shoulder joint.

Gradual conditioning: Gradually increase the intensity and duration of training to allow muscles, tendons, and joints to adapt to the demands of artistic swimming.

Warm-up and cooldown: Prioritize a thorough warm-up before training sessions and cooldown with stretching afterward to adapt muscles and joints for activity and help in recovery.

Listen to your body: Pay attention to any warning signs of pain or discomfort. If the pain persists and the range of motion is reduced, look for a professional, a sports medicine specialist [40].

7.12 Knee and Hip

Knee and hip injuries are relatively joint in artistic swimming due to the repetitive nature of the sport, as well as the strain placed on these joints during various maneuvers. Here is an overview of the diagnosis, treatment, and prevention of knee and hip injuries in artistic swimming:

Diagnosis and medical evaluation: It is important for the understanding of the symptoms to perform a medical history and an examination to evaluate the extent of the injury.

Imaging tests, like X-rays, magnetic resonance imaging (MRI), or ultrasound, may be used to get a detailed view of the joint and identify structural damage or abnormalities.

Joint knee and hip injuries: Patellofemoral pain syndrome involves pain around or behind the kneecap (patella) brought on by repetitive stress or improper alignment.

Meniscus tears: Twisting or rotational movements can lead to tears in the menisci, which are cartilage pads that cushion the knee joint.

Anterior cruciate ligament (ACL) tears: Sudden stops or direction changes can cause ACL tears, a crucial ligament stabilizing the knee.

Hip impingement: The femoral head and acetabulum (hip socket) can rub against each other, causing pain and potential cartilage damage.

The treatment is based on rest and immobilization. It depends on the severity of the injury; you may need to rest and limit weight-bearing activities to allow healing.

Physical therapy: Specific exercises can improve the strength, flexibility, and stability of the affected joint, promoting recovery and preventing further injury.

Medications: Nonsteroidal anti-inflammatory drugs (NSAIDs) may be prescribed to reduce pain and inflammation.

Surgical intervention: In severe cases, surgical procedures should be needed.

Prevention: Proper technique and training. Ensure you have proper coaching and training to learn the correct technique to reduce the risk of injury.

Conditioning and strengthening: Maintenance of a regular conditioning program, including exercises to strengthen the muscles around the knee and hip joints.

Warm-up and stretching: Before training or competition, perform warm-up exercises and stretching routines to prepare the muscles and joints for activity.

7.13 Lumbar Problems

Similar to other sports modalities, especially gymnastics, synchronized swimming significantly impacts the lumbar spine. Some technically necessary elements require a pronounced lumbar hyperextension. The underlying physiopathology of low back pain is still not unequivocally established. The commonly cited causes are facet joint inflammation, abdominal and hip flexor muscle weakness, incorrect pelvic posture, and repeated micro-traumatic action (overuse). The pain often can also result from a deficit in muscular control of the lumbar spine, particularly during the execution of specific fundamental technical movements at high speeds. In this sport, despite the prevalence of low back pain, it is not accompanied, in the majority of cases, by neurological signs [35]. The pain is provoked and exacerbated by activity, especially during hyperextension actions. The objective examination (physical examination) may include palpable spasm of the erector spinal muscle, evidence of facet joint inflammation during extension, tightness of the iliopsoas and quadriceps muscle groups, hypomobility of the spinal column, and abnormal lumbar and pelvic posture [35]. It is essential to rule out other causes of back pain, excluding the presence of bone, discogenic, or intra-abdominal pathologies. Radiological evaluation is likely to be negative.

Treatment for this injury should include education for the athlete and the coach. Modifying frequency, intensity, speed, and degree of hyperextension during the acute phase is necessary. Maximizing the flexibility of the surrounding musculature is essential, as well as strengthening the appropriate muscle groups to ensure spinal stabilization. Correction of postural abnormalities and hypomobility is recommended. The use of ice, anti-inflammatory medication, and physical therapy modalities such as heat therapy, ultrasound, and massage can also be beneficial in managing symptoms and promoting healing. It is important to gradually return to activity and sports participation, ensuring proper warm-up, stretching, and conditioning exercises are implemented. In conclusion, as in other sports, lumbar pathology in synchronized swimming can be attributed to various factors, including inflammation, muscle weakness, poor posture, and overuse. Proper diagnosis, treatment, and preventive measures are essential to manage low-back pain and promote artistic swimmers' overall well-being and performance.

This happens due to incorrect technique and excessive loads. You can also damage the lumbar region if the program is not initiated correctly or during weightlifting. And, of course, remember to constantly elevate your technique level, as there are numerous cases of pinched nerves in the lumbar region or pinched sciatic nerve—the sensations could be more pleasant.

The use of ice, anti-inflammatory medication, and physical therapy modalities such as heat therapy, ultrasound, and massage can also be beneficial in managing symptoms and promoting healing. It is important to gradually return to activity and sports participation, ensuring proper warm-up, stretching, and conditioning exercises are implemented.

In conclusion, lumbar pathology in artistic swimming, as in other sports, can be attributed to various factors, including inflammation, muscle weakness, poor posture, and overuse. Proper diagnosis, treatment, and preventive measures are essential to manage low-back pain and promote artistic swimmers' overall well-being and performance.

7.14 Neck Injuries

In artistic swimming, neck injuries can indeed occur, taking into account the movements involved in the sport. Here are some common neck injuries that can occur in artistic swimming:

Muscle strains: The repetitive lifting and turning of the head during routines can strain the neck muscles. This can happen when the muscles are overworked or subjected to excessive force. Muscle strains can cause pain, stiffness, and limited range of motion in the neck.

Muscle spasms: Intense or sudden movements in artistic swimming, especially when combined with fatigue or improper technique, can lead to muscle spasms in the neck. These spasms are involuntary contractions of the muscles and can cause severe pain and temporary loss of function.

Whiplash: Whiplash injuries can occur when the head and neck forcefully and rapidly move in opposite directions. Although less common in artistic swimming compared to contact sports, whiplash can still happen if a swimmer's head abruptly contacts the water's surface. Whiplash can result in neck pain, stiffness, headaches, and, in some cases, more severe symptoms.

To prevent neck injuries in artistic swimming, swimmers need to focus on proper technique, maintain good posture, and gradually build strength and flexibility in the neck and upper body muscles. Warm-up exercises that target the neck and shoulder areas can also help prepare the muscles for the demands of the sport. Additionally, using appropriate equipment, such as nose clips and goggles, can reduce the risk of sudden head movements and potential injuries. If a neck injury occurs, seeking medical attention and following appropriate treatment protocols, including rest, physical therapy, pain management, and rehabilitation exercises, are essential.

Return to play: As with any sport, injuries can occur in artistic swimming, and it's essential to approach the return-to-play process with caution to ensure the athlete's safety. Here are some general guidelines for returning to play after an injury in artistic swimming:

Medical evaluation: The first step is to consult with a medical professional, such as a sports medicine doctor or a physical therapist, who can assess and diagnose the injury's severity. They will develop an appropriate treatment plan and determine when returning to training is safe.

Rehabilitation: Following the medical evaluation, a rehabilitation program will be prescribed to aid recovery. This program may include exercises to restore strength, improve flexibility, and address any imbalances or weaknesses contributing to the injury.

Gradual progression: Returning to complete training or competition should be gradual. Athletes should start with light conditioning exercises and gradually increase the intensity and complexity of their training. This allows the body to adapt and reduces the risk of re-injury.

Technique and skill refinement: In artistic swimming, proper technique and execution of skills are crucial. Athletes must focus on refining their technique during the return-to-play process. Coaches should provide guidance and feedback to ensure that skills are performed correctly, reducing the risk of further injury.

Communication and monitoring: Athletes should communicate openly with their medical team, coaches, and support staff throughout the return-to-play process. Regular check-ins and progress evaluations will help ensure that the athlete is progressing safely and can make any necessary adjustments to their training plan.

Mental and emotional readiness: Besides physical readiness, athletes must be mentally and emotionally prepared to return to play. Injuries can take a toll on an athlete's confidence, so providing a supportive environment and allowing athletes to regain their trust in their abilities are essential.

Every injury is unique, and the return-to-play process should be tailored to the individual athlete's needs. Working closely with coaches and support staff ensures a safe return to artistic swimming.

7.15 Health Relationship Problems and Adequate Treatment

Combining intense physical activity, breathing control techniques, and exposure to allergenic products can sometimes result in respiratory problems such as exercise-induced asthma or bronchoconstriction.

While respiratory problems may not be as prevalent in artistic swimming as in other sports, there are still a few conditions that athletes in this discipline may encounter. Here are a few respiratory medical problems that can affect artistic swimmers [24]:

Asthma: Asthma is a respiratory condition affecting individuals involved in any sport, including artistic swimming. Airway inflammation and narrowing lead to respiratory symptoms such as wheezing, coughing, and shortness of breath. Swimmers with asthma should work closely with their healthcare providers to manage their condition and ensure optimal lung function.

Exercise-induced bronchoconstriction (EIB): Also known as exercise-induced asthma, EIB is a condition in which physical activity triggers the narrowing of the airways. It can cause symptoms like coughing, wheezing, chest tightness, and shortness of breath. Artistic swimmers may experience EIB during intense training sessions or performances (Fig. 7.4) due to physical exertion and exposure to chlorine or other irritants in the pool environment [16, 17].

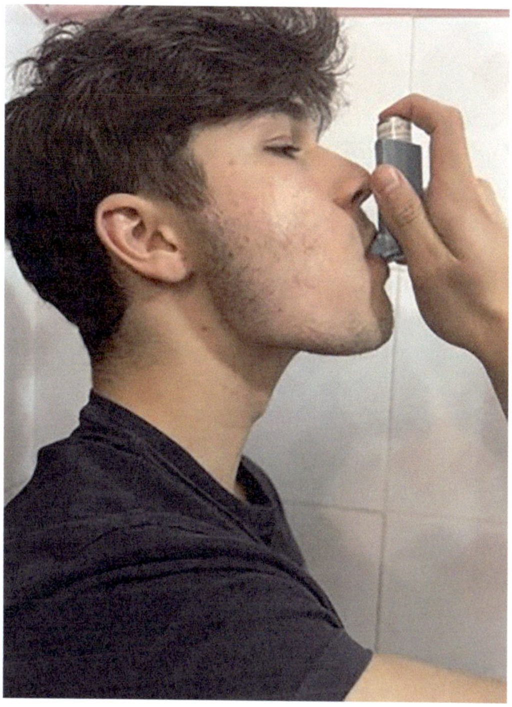

Fig. 7.4 Exercise-induced bronchoconstriction (EIB) may need therapeutic use of bronchodilators

Respiratory infections: Frequent exposure to water and close contact with other swimmers can increase the risk of respiratory infections, especially upper respiratory tract infections. These infections can cause symptoms like coughing, congestion, sore throat, and fatigue. Proper hygiene practices, including regular handwashing and avoiding swimming while sick, can help reduce the risk of respiratory infections.

Allergies: Some artistic swimmers may have allergies to substances in the pool environment, such as chlorine or other chemicals used for water treatment. Allergies can lead to respiratory symptoms like sneezing, runny nose, itchy eyes, and coughing. Swimmers with allergies should identify and avoid triggers whenever possible or seek appropriate medical treatment to manage their symptoms effectively.

To address respiratory issues and ensure the well-being of artistic swimmers, coaches, trainers, and athletes need to focus on proper warm-up and cooldown routines, maintain good indoor air quality in training facilities, encourage hydration, and promote overall respiratory health through appropriate conditioning exercises and breathing techniques. It is also crucial for athletes to consult with healthcare professionals to manage any pre-existing conditions or symptoms they may experience.

7.16 Mental Health

Like any high-performance sport, artistic swimming can exert significant mental and emotional pressure on athletes. Pursuing perfection, intense training schedules, and performance expectations can contribute to stress, anxiety, and other mental health issues.

It is essential for artistic swimmers to have access to proper medical care, including sports medicine professionals and specialists who understand the specific demands of their sport. Regular preventive measures, proper technical training, and a balanced lifestyle can help minimize the risk of problems and improve the overall well-being of artistic swimmers.

7.17 Ear, Eye, and Dermatologic Problems

Frequent exposure to water, especially in chlorinated pools, can make artistic swimmers more prone to ear infections, known as external otitis or "swimmer's ear." It occurs when water remains in the ear canal, creating a moist environment that facilitates the growth of bacteria or fungi [41].

Treatment and prevention of a swimmer's ear involve several measures. Here are some recommendations:

Keep the ears dry: After swimming or showering, gently dry the ears using a towel or a hairdryer on a low setting. Tilt your head to each side to allow water to drain out.

Avoid inserting objects into the ear: Refrain from using cotton swabs, bobby pins, or any other objects to clean the ear canal, as they can cause damage to the ear canal.

Use earplugs or a swim cap: Consider using earplugs designed explicitly for swimming to prevent water from entering the ear canal. Wearing a swim cap can also help keep the ears dry.

Use eardrops: Over-the-counter ear drops can help prevent swimmer's ears by drying out the ear canal or creating an acidic environment that discourages bacterial or fungal growth.

Avoid excessive cleaning: While keeping the ears clean is essential, avoid over-cleaning or using harsh products, which affect the natural balance of the ear canal, increasing the risk of infection.

If an ear infection develops, it is recommended to seek medical advice for appropriate treatment. Treatment may involve [41]:

Prescription eardrops: Your doctor may prescribe eardrops that contain antibiotics to fight bacterial infections or antifungal medication for fungal infections.

Pain relief: Acetaminophen or ibuprofen may be recommended to alleviate discomfort.

Ear cleaning: In some cases, your doctor may need to clean excessive earwax or debris from the ear canal to facilitate the effectiveness of eardrops.

7.18 Eye Problems

Artistic swimmers can experience ocular problems due to the nature of their sport. Some common ocular issues that artistic swimmers may encounter include:

Chlorine-related eye irritation: The chlorine used in swimming pools can cause eye irritation, dryness, and redness. This can be managed by wearing goggles designed for swimming to protect the eyes from direct contact with the water [42].

Corneal abrasions: these can occur when the cornea's surface gets scratched [43]. This can happen due to accidental contact with a partner's hand or foot during a routine. Immediate medical attention is required, and treatment may involve antibiotic eye drops or ointments to prevent infection and promote healing.

Dry eye syndrome: Dry eye can develop due to prolonged exposure to chlorine and other chemicals in pool water. Symptoms include dryness, itchiness, redness, and a gritty eye sensation. Over-the-counter artificial tears can help alleviate symptoms; in severe cases, prescription medications or eye inserts may be necessary.

To diagnose ocular problems, artistic swimmers should seek an evaluation from an ophthalmologist specializing in sports vision or eye care. These professionals can perform a comprehensive eye examination, assess specific issues, and recommend appropriate treatments [44].

Prevention is crucial in minimizing ocular problems in artistic swimmers. Here are some preventive measures:

Wearing goggles: Always wear well-fitted, swim-specific goggles to protect the eyes from irritants, chlorine, and potential trauma.

Regular eye breaks: During training sessions, take short breaks to rest the eyes, and allow them to recover from the chlorine and pool water exposure.

Proper hydration: Stay properly hydrated to help maintain tear film stability and prevent dry eye symptoms.

Eye hygiene: Maintain good eye hygiene by avoiding touching or rubbing the eyes with chlorine-contaminated hands.

Regular eye exams: Schedule regular eye examinations with an eye care professional to monitor eye health and detect potential issues early on.

Remember, consulting with a healthcare professional for accurate diagnosis, personalized treatment, and appropriate preventive measures based on individual circumstances is essential.

A few potential eye problems can occur in artistic swimming:

Chlorine-related issues: Artistic swimming pools are typically treated with chlorine to maintain water quality. Prolonged exposure to chlorine can cause eye problems such as irritation, redness, dryness, and, in some cases, even corneal abrasions.

Conjunctivitis: this is characterized by an inflammation of the thin, transparent layer covering the eye's white part and the eyelids' inner surface [43, 44]. Also known as "pink eye," bacterial or viral infections, allergies, or exposure to irritants like chlorine can cause it.

Contact lens–related issues: Some artistic swimmers wear contact lenses during performances. However, the chlorine in the water can cause lens discomfort, irritation, and even infections if proper hygiene practices are not followed.

7.19 Dermatological Problems

Dry skin and dermatitis can be common issues in artistic swimming; the nature of the sport, which involves spending a significant amount of time in chlorinated water, can lead to these skin problems [45]. To help manage dry skin and dermatitis in artistic swimming:

Moisturize: Use a good-quality moisturizer regularly to hydrate your skin and create a barrier against chlorine. Look for moisturizers that are fragrance-free and suitable for sensitive skin.

Shower before swimming: Rinse your body with fresh water before entering the pool.

Wear a swim cap: Wearing a swim cap reduces the amount of chlorine that comes into direct contact with your hair and scalp, contributing to dryness and dermatitis.

Rinse immediately after swimming: After each practice or performance, rinse off thoroughly with fresh water to remove any chlorine residue from your skin. Use a gentle cleanser if needed, but avoid harsh soaps that can further dry out your skin.

Avoid hot showers because they can strip your skin of its natural oils, exacerbating dryness. Stick to lukewarm water when showering.

Choose gentle skincare products: Option for gentle, fragrance-free cleansers and body washes that are specifically formulated for sensitive skin. Avoid products with alcohol or harsh chemicals that can further irritate your skin.

Hydrate: Drink plenty of water to guarantee that your body and skin stay hydrated.

Consult a dermatologist: A dermatologist can be very helpful. It is best to consult a dermatologist if you are experiencing persistent or severe dryness or dermatitis. They can provide personalized advice and recommend specific skin-care products or treatments to address your concerns.

As mentioned before, artistic swimming is a very demanding and complex sport. In this chapter, we have mentioned only some generalities concerning the physiology, injuries, and some common medical problems; each of these items mentioned should be specifically developed to allow research in order to know more and more about this fantastic sports discipline.

References

1. Mountjoy M. The basics of synchronized swimming and its injuries. Clin Sports Med. 1999;18(2):321–36. https://doi.org/10.1016/s0278-5919(05)70148-4.
2. Alentejano T, Bell G, Marshall D. A comparison of the physiological responses to underwater arm cranking and breath holding between synchronized swimmers and breath holding untrained women. J Hum Kinet. 2012;32:147–56.
3. Rodríguez-Zamora L, et al. Blood lactate accumulation during competitive freediving and synchronized swimming. Undersea Hyperb Med. 2018;45(1):55–63.
4. Mountjoy M. Injuries and medical issues in synchronized Olympic sports. Curr Sports Med Rep. 2009;8:255–61. https://doi.org/10.1249/JSR.0b013e3181b84a09.
5. Viana E, Bentley D, Logan-Sprenger HM. A physiological overview of the demands, characteristics, and adaptations of highly trained artistic swimmers: a literature review. Sports Med Open. 2019;5:16. https://doi.org/10.1186/s40798-019-0190-3.

6. Mountjoy M, et al. Sports injuries and illnesses in the 2009 FINA world championships (aquatics). Br J Sports Med. 2010;44(7):522–7.
7. Nakashima M, et al. Simulation analysis of lift in synchronized swimming. J Aero Aqua Bio-Mech. 2013;3(1):51–6.
8. FINA. FINA Artistic Swimming Rules 2017–2021. 2017 [cited 2018 April 23,2018]
9. Sydnor S. A history of synchronized swimming. J Sport History. 1998;25(2):252–67.
10. Roby FB, et al. Physiological characteristics of champion synchronized swimmers. Phys Sportsmed. 1983;11(4):136–47.
11. Rodríguez-Zamora L, et al. Physiological responses in relation to performance during competition in elite synchronized swimmers. PLoS One. 2012;7(11):e49098.
12. Rodríguez-Zamora L, et al. Monitoring internal load parameters during competitive synchronized swimming duet routines in elite athletes. J Strength Cond Res. 2014;28(3):742–51.
13. Rovnaya OA, Podrigalo LV, Aghyppo OY, Cieslicka M, Stankiewicz B. Study of functional potentials of different portsmanship level synchronous swimming sportswomen under impact of hypoxia. Res J Pharm Biol Chem Sci. 2016;7:1210–9.
14. Quan L, Culver BH, Fielding R. Hypoxia-induced loss of consciousness in multiple synchronized swimmers during a workout. Int J Aquatic Res Educ. 2010;4(4):5.
15. Podrihalo O, Podrigalo L, Jagiełło W, Iermakov S, Yermakova T. Substantiation of methods for predicting success in artistic swimming. Int J Environ Res Public Health. 2021;18(16):8739. https://doi.org/10.3390/ijerph18168739.
16. Figura F, Cama G, Guidetti L. Heart rate, alveolar gases and blood lactate during synchronized swimming. J Sports Sci. 1993;11(2):103–7.
17. García I, Drobnic F, Pons V, Viscor G. Changes in lung diffusing capacity of elite artistic swimmers during training. Int J Sports Med. 2021;42:227–33.
18. Naranjo J, et al. A test for evaluation of exercise with apneic episodes in synchronized swimming. Int J Sports Med. 2006;27(12):1000–4.
19. Ponciano K, et al. Physiological responses during the practice of synchronized swimming: a systematic review. Clin Physiol Funct Imaging. 2018;38(2):16.
20. Lundy B. Nutrition for synchronized swimming: a review. Int J Sport Nutr Exerc Metab. 2011;21(5):436–45.
21. Robertson S, Benardot D, Mountjoy M. Nutritional recommendations for synchronized swimming. Int J Sport Nutr Exerc Metab. 2014;24(4):404–13.
22. Auer RN, Sutherland G. Hypoxia and related conditions. Greenfield's Neuropathol. 2002;1:233–80.
23. Yamamura S, Zushi K, Takata T, Ishiko N, Matsui KK. Physiological characteristics of well-trained synchronized swimmers in relation to performance scores. Int J Sports Med. 1999;20(4):246–51.
24. Andersson J, et al. Cardiovascular and respiratory responses to apneas with and without face immersion in exercising humans. J Appl Physiol. 2004;96(3):1005–10.
25. Kjeld T, et al. Release of erythropoietin and neuron-specific enolase after breath holding in competing free divers. Scand J Med Sci Sports. 2015;25
26. Davies B, Donaldson G, Joels N. Do the competition rules of synchronized swimming encourage undesirable levels of hypoxia? Br J Sports Med. 1995;29(1):16–9.
27. Jamnik V, et al. An evaluation of the physiological response to competitive synchronized swimming and the physiological characteristics of elite synchronized swimmers. Toronto: York University; 1987.
28. Bante S, et al. Cardiorespiratory and metabolic responses to a simulated synchronized swimming routine in senior (> 18 years) and comen (13-15 years) national level athletes. J Sports Med Phys Fitness. 2007;47(3):291.
29. Rodríguez FA, Mader A. Energy systems in swimming. In: World book of swimming: from science to performance, vol. 11; 2011. p. 225.
30. Alentejano TC, Marshall D, Bell GJ. Breath holding with water immersion in synchronized swimmers and untrained women. Res Sports Med. 2010;18(2):97–114.
31. Gemma KE, Wells CL. Heart rates of elite synchronized swimmers. Phys Sportsmed. 1987;15(10):99–107.
32. Bentley DJ, Viana E, Logan-Sprenger HM. Metabolic and performance responses to a simulated routine in elite artistic swimmers. Sports. 2022;10:190. https://doi.org/10.3390/sports101201.
33. Junge A, Engebretsen L, Mountjoy ML, Alonso JM, Renström PA, Aubry MJ, Dvorak J. Sports injuries during the summer Olympic games 2008. Am J Sports Med. 2009;37(11):2165–72. https://doi.org/10.1177/0363546509339357.
34. McCrory P, Meeuwisse W, Johnston K, et al. Zurich consensus statement on concussion in sport. Clin J Sport Med. 2009;19:185–200.
35. Dyrek D, Micheli L, Magee D. Injuries to the thoracolumbar spine and pelvis. In: Zachazewski J, Magee D, Quillen W, editors. Athletic injuries and rehabilitation. Philadelphia: WB Saunders; 1996. p. 465–85.
36. Mountjoy M. The basics in synchronized swimming and its injuries. Clin Sport Med. 1999;18:321–36.
37. Mountjoy M, Gerrard D. Preserving and promoting health in the aquatic athlete. In: Seifert L, Chollet D, Mujika I, editors. World book of swimming: from science to performance. Hauppauge: Nova Science Publishers.
38. Mountjoy M, Junge A, Alonso JM, Clarsen B, Pluim BM, Shrier I, van den Hoogenband C, Marks S, Gerrard D, Heyns P, Kaneoka K, Dijkstra HP, Khan KM. Consensus statement on the methodology of injury and illness surveillance in FINA (aquatic

sports). Br J Sports Med. 2016;50(10):590–6. https://doi.org/10.1136/bjsports-2015-095686.
39. McCrory P, Meeuwisse W, Dvorak J, Aubry M, Bailes J, Broglio S, et al. Consensus statement on concussion in sport – the 5th international conference on concussion in sport held in Berlin, October 2016. Br J Sports Med. 2017;51(11):838–47.
40. Tovin BJ. Prevention and treatment of swimmer's shoulder. N Am J Sports Phys Ther. 2006;1(4):166–75.
41. Wang MC, Liu CY, Shiao AS, Wang T. Ear problems in swimmers. J Chin Med Assoc. 2005;68(8):347–52. https://doi.org/10.1016/S1726-4901(09)70174-1.
42. Skeldon S. Red eye in sports. Br J Sports Med. 2018;52(5):305–6.
43. Hitti W, Abdelmassih Y. Acute conjunctivitis in athletes: a review. Sports Med. 2016;46(10):1451–60.
44. Solomon A, Lindsley K. Conjunctivitis: a systematic review of diagnosis and treatment. JAMA. 2017;317(19):1931–43.
45. Freiman A, Barankin B, Elpern DJ. Sports dermatology part 2: swimming and other aquatic sports. CMAJ. 2004;171(11):1339–41. https://doi.org/10.1503/cmaj.1040892.

8 Artistic Roller Skating

Carolina A. Cabo

8.1 Introduction

Skating is an activity that involves moving, or sliding, over a surface. It includes several disciplines that can be practiced on ice, as well as on synthetic or wooden sidewalk, with roller skates [1].

The 1908 Olympic Games in London were the first to include skating in its program. It consists in describing figures, jumping, pirouetting, etc. It is practiced in three modalities: individual, pairs, and dance. Historically, ice skating preceded the emergence of roller skates since the invention of ice skates was a necessity of daily life in countries with colder climates. Only secondarily was their use in sports [2]. For the times when ice was lacking, the use of proper skates, equipped with wheels instead of blades, emerged as an alternative, to enable the practice of the sport during the summer.

World skating is the body that regulates the various skating disciplines worldwide [3] and the Federação Portuguesa de Patinagem is the body that regulates the various skating disciplines at national level [4].

Skating is a sports modality, which implies a high demand on the part of the practitioner on a physical and mental level, in order to achieve adequate mastery of the techniques and their improvement to levels that can be presented in public [5].

Skating is a fitness sport for life, suitable for both children and adults. It helps improve cardiovascular fitness, as well as balance and coordination. As a sport, it requires efficient speed, balance, power, strength, endurance, coordination, and agility [6, 7]. It can also promote social adaptability in children and adolescents [8].

The skating federation is composed of the following disciplines: roller freestyle (RF), rink hockey (RH), artistic roller skating (ARS), speed skating (SS), skateboarding (SK), and inline freestyle (IF). This federation has a total of 16,077 registered athletes and a total of 270 clubs in different sports. The athletes are divided by their respective disciplines as follows: 12 RF; 6524 RH; 8417 ARS; 723 SS; 272 SK; and 129 IF, with ARS being the modality with the largest number of athletes [4].

C. A. Cabo (✉)
Departamento de Desporto e Saúde, Escola de Saúde e Desenvolvimento Humano, Universidade de Évora, Évora, Portugal

Comprehensive Health Research Centre (CHRC), Universidade de Évora, Évora, Portugal

Instituto Politécnico de Setúbal, Escola Superior de Educação, Setúbal, Portugal

Sport Physical Activity and Health Research & Innovation Center (SPRINT), Rio Maior, Portugal

H. Jones, A. Lukaszenko (eds.), *Injury Prevention and Care in Artistic Sports*,
https://doi.org/10.1007/978-3-032-18105-3_8

Artistic roller skating is considered an evolving sport that has been gaining more and more fans in recent years [9], especially children and adolescents.

Most skaters are female; in 2022, there were 8007 federated female athletes and only 410 federated male athletes in artistic roller skating. The beginning of the practice of figure skating is usually between 5 and 8 years old. They typically reach their career peak at puberty, before age 20 [10]. As we can prove with data from the Portuguese Skating Federation, in 2022, the largest number of athletes is in the 11–15 age group and tends to decrease in the succeeding age groups [4].

Despite having little recognition at national and international level, the growing number of active athletes from 2010 (3268 athletes) to 2020 (7666 athletes) has doubled. That number continues to increase to this day, having registered a total of 8417 federated figure-skating athletes in 2022 [4]. This exponential increase in athletes has made figure skating a highly competitive sport. High performance demands and rigorous and intense training are normally associated with this sport, which can lead to an increased risk of injuries [10].

As a significant number of young people experience increased training intensity, stresses on the dynamics of skeletal growth and muscle development are issues that may arise and deserve investigation [11]. Some studies have shown that skating can stimulate smaller muscles and joints and play a positive role in the balanced development of different parts of the body [8].

However, although artistic roller skating helps improve the health of athletes through exercise, it puts children at particular risk for injury [12]. Future injuries may be associated with recurring problems, such as acute or chronic, and appear to be common in artistic roller skating.

The main objective of this chapter is to describe what artistic roller skating is, what the participation habits are, and the most common physical complaints (PC) and injuries that arise in artistic roller skating.

8.2 Specificities of Sport/Artistic Roller Skating

Artistic roller skating is a sport based on an unnatural act, such as skating. As it is a cyclic action of propulsion, using instruments called roller skates, it is extremely important in the first approaches, the acquisition of static and dynamic balance in the correct placement of supports, and, at the beginning of propulsion, to know how to correctly provoke the body imbalances responsible for displacement [5].

It is a sport that encompasses a great technical complexity and a demanding artistic ability, which helps improve cardiovascular conditioning, as well as balance and coordination. As a sport, it requires efficient speed, balance, strength, power, endurance, coordination, and agility. This is a modality that combines technique, precision, balance, prowess, and aesthetics in perfect harmony with music. A modality of great beauty is the blend of sport and art whose competition can be individual and/or in pairs [7, 13].

8.2.1 Specialties

Artistic roller skating consists essentially of technical execution, interpretive and representational adaptation, and mastery of the roller skates. This activity has many specialties, such as:

- Free skating: Performed with individually choreographed music. It is characterized by leaps, spins, and steps, executed in a free and creative way, which gives it great spectacularism. The roller skater's virtuosity is defined by the speed, height of the jumps, number of rotations on the top, originality, difficulty, and safety in the connecting steps.
- Compulsory figures: Performed individually, without music. The athlete is asked to follow the circumferences previously traced in the ring with the roller skate. Performance assessment in mandatory figures is based on the figure's stroke, movement, and posture.

- Solo dance: Solo dance is very similar to pairs dance, with the particularity of being performed individually. It is a branch of skating that is on the rise and calls for beauty and spectacle.
- Artistic pairs: The pair is made up of a female element and a male element. Artistic Pairs are distinguished by the execution of jumps, tops, and elevations. The pair must work in harmony with the music, performing original movements.
- Dance pairs: The pair is made up of a female element and a male element. The pair's performances may include dance steps and balancing figures, but the athletes never break contact with each other. In dance pairs, there is an obligation to roller skate specific rhythms such as Waltz, Tango, Blues, Polka, Samba, Jive, etc. There is also free dance where the pair chooses their music and can explore their dancing and expression capacity to the fullest.
- Show and precision: The show is divided into quartets, small groups, and large groups. It is a unique competition where the teams combine their skills on roller skates with the dramatization of a small plot. Precision skating is distinguished by teamwork where the elements are completely synchronized in the formation of lines, wheels, bars, and blocks.

8.3 Epidemiology of More Frequent Injuries

In addition to understanding skating, it is also important to understand that the human body has many different anatomical structures and systems and different functions and that it is all subject to injury. An injury is characterized by structural damage to one or more system components, resulting in diminished functional capacity. All people have tissues that are susceptible to injury; this is due to inherent weakness or biomechanical factors. The risk of chronic injury in sport is then high, as specific repetitive movements are made in all of them.

Investigating the etiology of sports injuries, as well as implementing effective preventive measures, will allow to reduce not only the number of occurrences but also the events related to recurrences, the duration of the injury impact, and the underlying economic burden [14, 15].

Skating, in addition to improving the health of athletes through exercise, also exposes children to a risk of injury [12]. The mean age of starting the practice is 7.5 years, which is consistent with the findings by different authors [10, 16] that young people start practicing this modality very early, around 5–8 years, and reach the peak of their competitive career in adolescence or early adolescence.

Adolescents are more vulnerable to sports injuries because they participate earlier and more intensively in sports and in rapid growth and neurobiological maturation in an increasingly competitive and selective psychosocial environment. The pattern of injury occurrence (types, causes and distribution) in young adolescents is similar to that of adult professional athletes. In the young athlete still in the process of growth/development (particularly rapid in the pubertal jumping or "spurt period"), the growth cartilages at the ends of the long bones (epiphyses) are particularly vulnerable to mechanical overload injuries (compression forces) [17].

Another feature of these ages (10–16/17 years) that is a vulnerable point is related to the different rates of accelerated growth among bones, muscles, and ligaments. The peak of bone growth is out of phase (before) the peak of soft tissue growth. This increases the susceptibility to injury at the bony attachment sites of tendons and ligaments. On the other hand, the rhythms of growth and neurobiological maturation are individual and determined by the interaction between genetic and environmental factors [17]. Since the division by age groups in all sports is made exclusively by chronological age, two youngsters with the same chronological age may have different maturational profiles [18].

The level of competitiveness and the varied specialties within artistic figure skating mean that athletes have to push themselves as hard as possible in training to achieve the minimum requirements needed to participate in competitions that occur throughout the year, which, according to Fortin and Roberts [19], increases vulnerability to injury occurrence.

The sport that presents the highest risk of injury is individual artistic roller skating, due to the high number of vertical jumps, figures, various body positions, and spinning tops. Vertical jumps happen with the vertical projection of the body in rotation, and their landing occurs only on one of the lower limbs. The body positions and figures require a lot of motor skill, flexibility, and proprioception and are part of the choreography between a jumping element and a spinning element (not necessarily in this order). These positions and figures constitute stipulated elements that the athletes must perform during the choreography and remain for a period of time stipulated by the competition rules, and only then be scored in the final score. The tops are made only on one leg, on which the athlete, standing or moving, performs as many rotations as possible with his/her supporting foot, always in contact with the ground [20].

In terms of training load per week, most roller skaters trained between 2 and 10 h in the past 12 months (84.0%). Within this interval of training hours, 62 (43.3%) trained between 5 and 10 h, while 58 (40.6%) trained between 2 and 5 h per week. Eighteen (12.6%) reported training less than 2 h and five (3.5%) more than 10 h per week [16] (Fig. 8.1).

During the preparation for a tournament, the training hours were adjusted. We analyze the behavior within each category and find that 60 (52.6%) roller skaters maintained their training load despite preparing for a competition, while 46 (40.4%) roller skaters followed the opposite approach and increased their training load [16].

The number of workouts per week showed significant differences with PC. Those who train for 5–10 h have more PC (50.7%). When we increase the number of hours, the number of PC tends to increase, but when we exceed 10 h, this does not happen, with only 7.5% of athletes indicating this value. Training above average can also raise the precondition since the musculoskeletal system is more willing to that load. Thus, we assume that

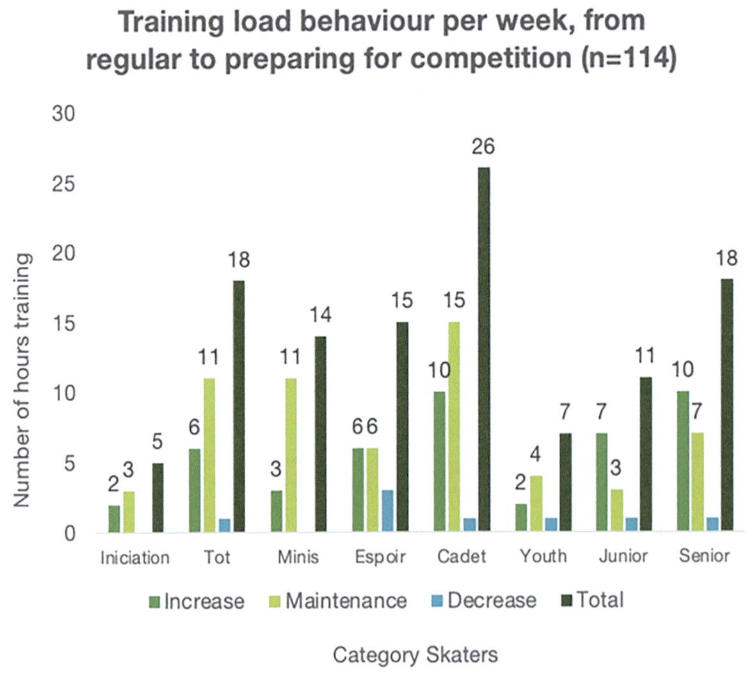

Fig. 8.1 Weekly training hours [16]

they have been practicing for over 10 h for several years. Hence, there is no oscillation [21].

Thus, training hours may increase the prevalence of injuries and physical complaints (PC), either in a regular training regime or in specific phases of preparation for particular events or championships [10].

Regarding the material, roller skaters maintained their wheels and bearings monthly (44.8%) or whenever they exhibited problems (32.9%). A smaller percentage (13.3%) was found among those who used a weekly maintenance schedule. The most common time periods for roller skate replacement were over 3 years (48.3%) and within 1–2 years (38.5%). Fewer roller skaters replaced their artistic roller skates annually (13.3%). Most roller skaters replaced their roller plates within 3 or more years (65.7%), followed by those who replaced every 1–2 years (32.9%). Only two roller skaters (1.4%) replaced their plates annually [16] (Fig. 8.2).

Wheels/bearings are not significant for chronic conditions, previous injuries, and PC. Boots have significant differences concerning PC. Those who change boots after three or more years are at a greater risk (58.2%); thus, the ability of boots to stabilize the ankle is relevant. About roller plates, there are significant differences in chronic conditions, with a greater number of those who change chassis after three or more years (83.4%) [21].

Thus, when a sports shoe is not suited to an individual's specific needs, it can cause movement patterns that overload the human locomotor structure, resulting in chronic pain and injury [22]. Furthermore, as a high-performance sport, skating requires hours of daily training and practice with an uncomfortable roller skate, which can cause injuries to the athlete's feet and impair their performance.

Boots have become increasingly stiffer over the last 20 years to accommodate the stress placed on them when performing triple and

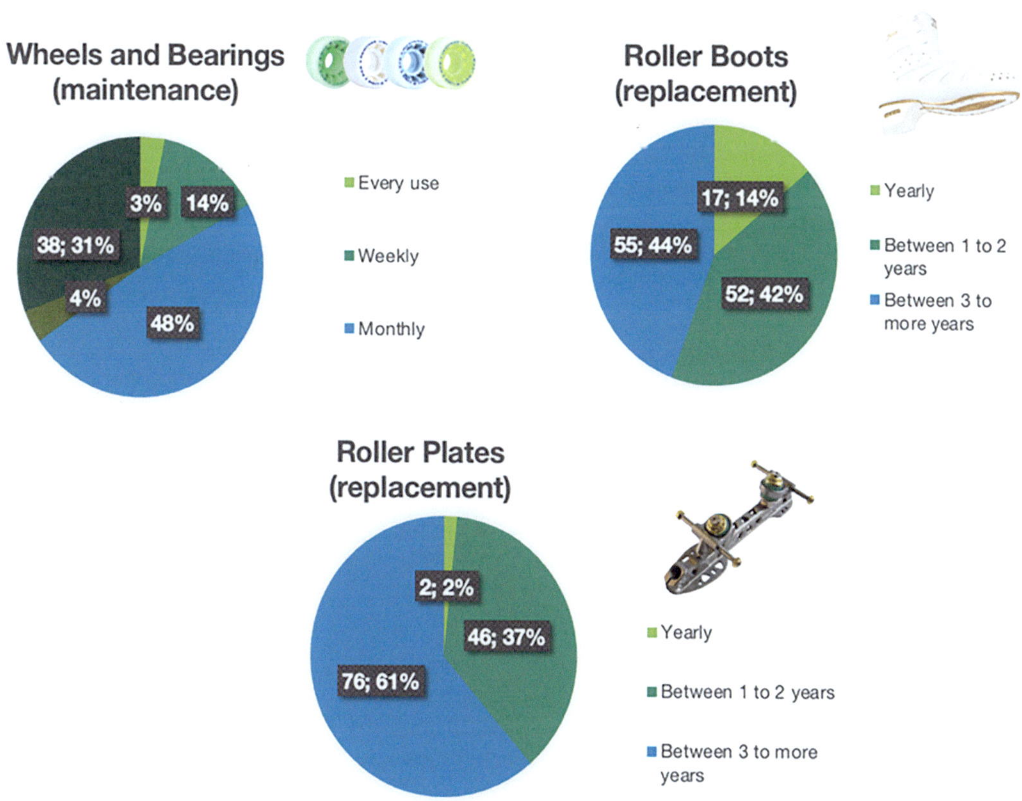

Fig. 8.2 Equipment [16]

quadruple jumps. It has been hypothesized that increased boot stiffness has contributed to weaker ankles in competitive roller skaters. The ankle is a common area of injury for artistic roller skaters. In a 2003 study of over 200 nationally competitive artistic roller skaters, 27.7% of the injuries reported on a medical history report involved the ankle, making it the most commonly affected body part [10].

Sixty-seven (46.9%) roller skaters reported PC in the past 12 months. The mean age was 14.24 years (range 7–24 years). A total of 175 PC were reported by these participants. The anatomical distribution was predominantly in the lower limbs (53.1%), followed by the trunk (24.0%) and upper limbs (22.9%) [16] (Fig. 8.3).

Artistic roller skating is a fast sport, but with good control. This may explain why roller skaters had more soft tissue injuries and dislocations. All roller skaters have a great tendency to cushion falls with their arms, and so much of the injuries occur in the upper extremity. About 87.5% of the fractures involved the upper limb, particularly the wrist [23].

From the sporting point of view, Gantus and Assumpção (2002) point out as main causes of injury the absence of preventive measures, competitive exhaustion, athletic voluptuousness, and psychosomatism [20].

Common problems in artistic figure skating include acute musculoskeletal injuries, chronic overuse injuries, and medical problems. Contributing factors are the training regime, environmental factors, and conventions of the sport that reward high-risk movements. Studies have shown that about 50% of injuries are traumatic and 50% are due to an overuse mechanism. Overuse injuries are more common in individual roller skaters, while acute injuries are more common in pair skaters. The difference is likely due to throws in pair and dance skaters, which increases speed, momentum, and force in falls and injury severity. It is estimated that 50–78% of injuries are preventable [10].

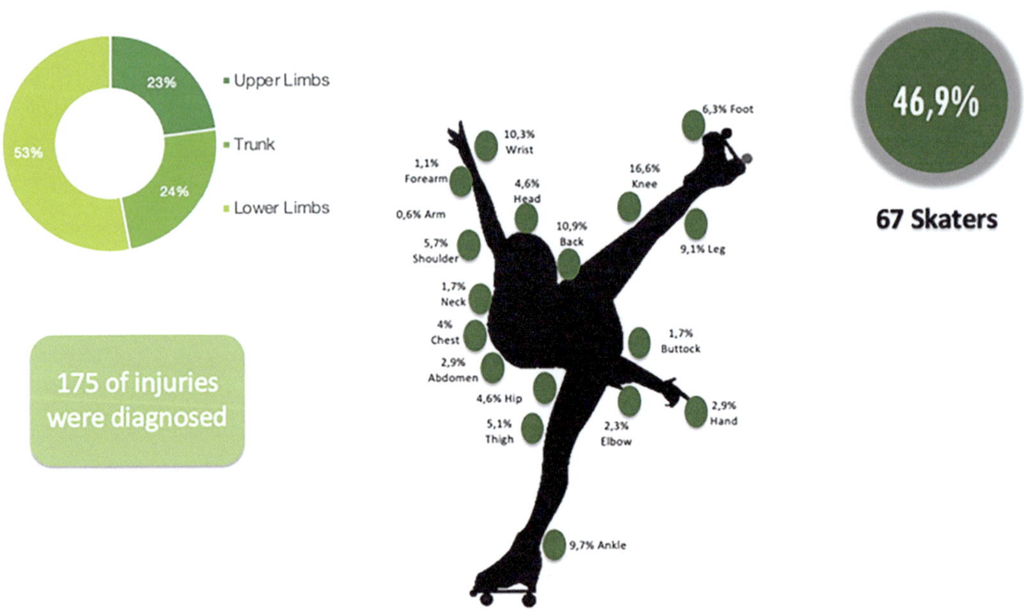

Fig. 8.3 Distribution of PC per anatomical distribution of PC [16]

8.4 Diagnosis, Treatment Options, and Return to Performance

The risk of injury will always be inevitably associated with any sports activity due to its nature, but we can reduce it if we achieve a greater knowledge about the subject and how to carry out effective preventive work [24]. We'll take a deeper look at three of the most common areas of PC in artistic roller skating, the low back, ankle, and knee (Fig. 8.4).

Low-back pain can be caused by lumbar strains, facet pain, posterior iliac crest injurics, spondylosis, or spondylolisthesis. These injuries can be related to the stiffness of the roller skater's boot. Increased stiffness limits ankle and knee motion, causing the roller skater to increase flexion in the hip and extend the back to maintain balance. Dysfunction of the sacroiliac joint is also a common problem due to repeated unilateral loads and shear forces [10].

Evaluation of low-back pain should include radiological imaging to rule out congenital etiologies, spondylosis, spondylolisthesis, and stress fractures [10].

Treatment of lower-back problems should include physical therapy and exercises to strengthen the core muscles of the roller skater to protect the spine.

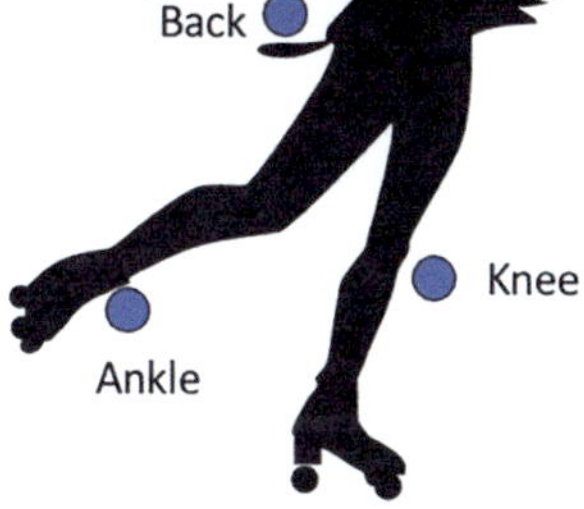

Fig. 8.4 The most common areas of PC [21]

Ankle sprain is a common injury because artistic roller skaters have relatively weak peroneal muscles, most of which result from the inversion movement, and the most affected ligament is the anterior peroneal-talar joint. A less common mechanism of injury involves a strong eversion movement injuring the deltoid ligament complex (on the medial aspect of the ankle). In roller skaters, ankle sprains usually occur during off-track training sessions. To prevent these injuries, roller skaters should incorporate ankle stabilization and proprioceptive training into their off-track training [10].

Ankle sprain consists of pain, discomfort, heat, and/or swelling located on the lateral side, immediately in front of the ankle; bruising on the lateral aspect, immediately in front of the ankle, which may spread to the rest of the dorsum of the foot and toes, depending on the severity of the injury; difficulty walking/putting the foot on the ground; and/or characteristic gait pattern [10].

All of these symptoms can vary in intensity, depending on the severity of the sprain. Sometimes, pain and swelling are absent in people with a history of sprain. Instead, you may simply feel your ankle unstable when you walk. Still, treatment is crucial.

For ankle injuries, there are four phases to rehabilitation, a first phase of rest, elevation of the ankle, ice, anti-inflammatory medications, and immobilization for 6–12 weeks until pain and swelling improve; a second phase in which support and gait training begins, with supervised motor physiotherapy to improve ankle movement and increase strength and muscle stability; a third phase in which we intensify strength and proprioception training; and a fourth phase with rapid changes in direction, jumping and braking [25].

After a lateral ligamentous injury, it is difficult to predict precisely when the athlete can return to sports (RTS). Furthermore, residual disability of ankle joint sprains is often caused by an inadequate rehabilitation program and early RTS [25].

Continuing sport-specific rehabilitation will help minimize this risk. The time needed to RTS in lateral ligamentous ankle sprains depends on several factors, including the severity of the injury, the ability of the athlete, and the rehabilitation features available [25].

Tendonitis in the knee consists of an inflammation of the tendon, which can be in the quadriceps tendon or the rotulian tendon. The most common symptoms are pain, lack of strength in the knee, swelling, and/or redness.

After a knee injury, proper strengthening of the quadriceps muscles and all those involving the tendons is necessary to resume performance. Strengthening exercises should be performed with the help of a trampoline, TheraBand, and weights. Ice should be applied in early stages or electrotherapy techniques to decrease inflammatory signs.

After an injury, it is necessary, in order to resume performance, depending on the severity of the injury, to analyze an athlete's ability to resume sports activities, all functional limitations arising from the damage must be restored, cardiovascular conditioning must be equal to or greater than the state pre-injury, and there should be no apprehension by the athlete or other members of the rehabilitation team regarding the safety of the athlete's health. The use of functional performance tests is considered useful for assessing the ability to perform sport-specific athletic skills again [25].

The planning process for resuming activity should incorporate forms of effort recovery, adequate nutritional intake, alternating training of the different activity components, and recognition of indicators that tell us that the physiological and psychological limits are being tested [17]. In general, a team approach including the skater, coach, parents, and physician, with the addition of an athletic trainer, physical therapist, nutritionist, sports psychologist, and orthopedist as needed, will help ensure the healthiest skaters [16].

8.5 Prevention

Injury prevention is mostly done by proper training and the use of preventive equipment. The use of protections such as the wrist, elbow, and knee pads, among others, should be considered.

8.6 Conclusion

Artistic figure skating PC are frequent. The number of workouts per week, the increase in training time, and the lack of material renewal are the most likely to present PC.

The most prevalent injuries are musculoskeletal injuries and repetitive strain injuries such as posterior tibial tendinopathy, generalized tendinitis, patellofemoral joint dysfunction, ankle and knee injuries, and leg injuries.

Factors that contribute to these injuries are roller skate, training regimen, environmental factors, and highly competitive sports.

The highest number of reports of injuries or PC are observed in the knees, followed by the back (mainly in the lumbar region) and ankles.

In practice, this study is essential so that coaches, trainers, physicists, and the entire multidisciplinary team that works with these athletes can improve their work, considering that participation habits will influence the appearance of PC and the number of them. It can often not be avoided but work to reduce the risk. In this way, there must be a complementary training without roller skates for strengthening of all muscles indicated as the most affected, to avoid increasing numbers of PC.

References

1. Cabo C. Queixas físicas e lesões relacionadas com a prática de Patinagem artística em Portugal: Um estudo epidemiológico [Universidade de Évora]. https://dspace.uevora.pt/rdpc/bitstream/10174/25794/1/Mestrado-Exerc%C3%ADcio_e_Sa%C3%BAde-Carolina_Alexandra_Alipio_Mourato_do_Cabo-Queixas_f%C3%ADsicas_e_les%C3%B5es_relacionadas_com_a_pr%C3%A1tica_de_patinagem....pdf (2019)
2. Formenti F, Minetti AE. Human locomotion on ice: the evolution of ice-skating energetics through history. J Exp Biol. 2007;210(10):1825–33. https://doi.org/10.1242/jeb.002162.
3. World Skate. World Skate. https://www.worldskate.org/ (2023)
4. FPP. FPP – Relatório e Contas 2022. https://fpp.pt/wp-content/uploads/RC_2022.pdf (2022)
5. Lagoa, M. Em busca do valor estético da ginástica artística feminina, da patinagem artística, do râguebi e do boxe: Estudo exploratório a partir da opinião

de treinadores. https://repositorio-aberto.up.pt/handle/10216/94466 (2009)

6. Ferrara CM, Hollingsworth E. Physical characteristics and incidence of injuries in adult figure skaters. Int J Sports Physiol Perform. 2007;2(3):282–91. https://doi.org/10.1123/ijspp.2.3.282.
7. Sehgal S, Esht V. Talent development of roller skating using an exercise program in young males: a study protocol for randomized controlled trial. Phys Ther Rev. 2019;24(6):6. https://doi.org/10.1080/10833196.2019.1648727.
8. Zhao W, Wang C, Hou L. Roller skating promotes the physical health of children and adolescents: a systematic review and meta analysis [Preprint]. In Review. https://doi.org/10.21203/rs.3.rs-85702/v1 (2020)
9. Lime Survey.: Lime Survey. http://www.limesurvey.org (2013)
10. Porter EB, Young CC, Niedfeldt MW, Gottschlich LM. Sport-specific injuries and medical problems of figure skaters. WMJ. 2007;106(6):6.
11. Stricker PR, Faigenbaum AD, McCambridge TM. Resistance training for children and adolescents. Pediatrics. 2020;145(6):e20201011. https://doi.org/10.1542/peds.2020-1011.
12. Knox CL, Comstock RD, McGeehan J, Smith GA. Differences in the risk associated with head injury for pediatric ice skaters, roller skaters, and inline skaters. Pediatrics. 2006;118(2):549–54. https://doi.org/10.1542/peds.2005-2913.
13. FPP. FPP PA – Plataforma. http://partistico.pt/Documentos/documentos1.php?dir=/Arquivo/2019 (2019)
14. Brooks JHM, Fuller CW. The influence of methodological issues on the results and conclusions from epidemiological studies of sports injuries: illustrative examples. Sports Med. 2006;36(6):459–72. https://doi.org/10.2165/00007256-200636060-00001.
15. van Mechelen W, Hlobil H, Kemper HCG. Incidence, severity, aetiology and prevention of sports injuries: a review of concepts. Sports Med. 1992;14(2):82–99. https://doi.org/10.2165/00007256-199214020-00002.
16. Cabo CA, Sousa JP, Bravo J. Participation habits, physical complaints and injuries in a sample of Portuguese female artistic roller skaters. Cultura, Ciencia y Deporte. 2022;17(54) https://doi.org/10.12800/ccd.v17i54.1879.
17. Oliveira R. Lesões nos Jovens Atletas: Conhecimento dos factores de risco para melhor prevenir. Revista Portuguesa de Fisioterapia no Desporto. 2007:33–8.
18. Jorna C, Elferink-Gemser MT. Effects of maturation on potential predictors of talent in soccer. In: e Silva MJC, Figueiredo AJ, Elferink-Gemser MT, Malina RM, editors. Youth sports: growth, maturation and talent. 1st ed. Imprensa da Universidade de Coimbra; 2016. p. 127–50. https://doi.org/10.14195/978-989-26-1169-3_9.
19. Fortin JD, Roberts D. Competitive figure skating injuries. Pain Physician. 2003;6(3):3.
20. dos Hoffmann, IS, Toigo AM. PREVALÊNCIA DE LESÕES MUSCULOESQUELÉTICAS EM ATLETAS AMADORES DE PATINAÇÃO ARTÍSTICA FEDERADOS NO ESTADO DO RIO GRANDE DO SUL (2016)
21. Cabo CA, Sousa JP, Bravo J. Physical complaints and participation habits in female artistic roller skaters. RETOS. 2023;48:775–83.
22. Wang I-L, Graham RB, Bourdon EJP, Chen Y-M, Gu C-Y, Wang L-I. Biomechanical analysis of running foot strike in shoes of different mass. J Sports Sci Med. 2020;19(1):130–7.
23. Horner C, McCabe MJ. Ice-skating and roller disco injuries in Dublin. Br J Sports Med. 1984;18(3):207–11. https://doi.org/10.1136/bjsm.18.3.207.
24. Muñoz D, Toro-Román V, Escudero-Tena A, Martínez BJS-A. Epidemiología de las lesiones laborales en entrenadores de pádel Epidemiology of occupational injuries in padel coaches. RETOS. 2023:359–64.
25. D'Hooghe P, Cruz F, Alkhelaifi K. Return to play after a lateral ligament ankle sprain. Curr Rev Musculoskelet Med. 2020;13(3):281–8. https://doi.org/10.1007/s12178-020-09631-1.

Figure Skating in Ice

9

A. Korolev, D. Ilyin, R. Ryazantsev, N. Magnitskaya, Z. Pilipson, R. Zaripov, and A. Logvinov

9.1 Introduction

Figure skating has come a long way, since the foundation of ISU in 1892, from sliding on ice and magnificent figures by Nikolai Panin (the first Olympic games champion, 1908) to modern figure skating, performed by individuals or pairs, with full of sophisticated elements—jumps, spins, lifts, and step sequences. Classical and the least traumatic figures on ice, such as circles, figures of eight, and many other elements, first described in 1772 by British figure skater Robert Jones, were performed till the end of the nineteenth century. Eventually, the elements became more complex, and these school figures were introduced in the international competitions till 1989. Nowadays, they are performed in step sequences. Figure skating jumps, characterized by high traumatism, were introduced from the end of the nineteenth century till 1920–1930. Axel, considered to be one of the most complex classical jumps, was first executed by Alex Paulsen in the 1880s. At the men's single competitions, this element was performed in the beginning of twentieth century and at the women's in the 1920s. Till the 1960s, only single and double jumps were performed. Vern Taylor was the first to execute triple Axel at the international competitions in 1978. The quadruple Axel, for a long time considered impossible, has been landed by Ilia Malinin. Nowadays, in ISU competitions, up to five quadruple jumps are accomplished in the free skating program. Over the years, figure skating gets more and more complex and potentially more traumatic.

9.2 Specifications

Figure skating is one of the most popular and traumatic ice sports. A lot of experience is needed to show thoughtful plasticity and grace on the ice. Ice skating involves a lot of complicated movement on blades of skates. In addition, there are a large number of jumps that need to be done artistically. Professionalism in jumping is a combination of execution technique and appropriate speed. Greater force is needed to push off and land. That is why achieving professional skating skills is more difficult than a basic level. This sport is associated with frequent falls, especially during competitions [1, 2]. Overload injuries prevail in single skating, which is associated with the growing technical complexity of the elements. In partner disciplines, acute injuries are more common, associated with a large number of throws and lifts with a high risk of falling [1, 3].

A. Korolev (✉) · D. Ilyin · R. Ryazantsev
N. Magnitskaya · Z. Pilipson · R. Zaripov
A. Logvinov
Olymp Clinic MARS and RUDN University of Russia Ersity, Peoples' Friendship University of Russia, Moscow, Russia

H. Jones, A. Lukaszenko (eds.), *Injury Prevention and Care in Artistic Sports*,
https://doi.org/10.1007/978-3-032-18105-3_9

9.3 Epidemiology of More Frequent Injuries

Epidemiology of figure skating injuries is variable and depends on the particular discipline. However, up to 80% of professional figure skaters sustained a traumatic event during their career. According to Fortin, the most common injuries occur during pair skating, single skating, and ice dancing [4]. Acute injuries predominantly occur in pair skaters (Fig. 9.1), synchronized skaters, and ice dancing, whereas overuse injuries occur in single skaters [1]. Also, it was noted that the amount of double, triple, and quadruple jumps in elite figure skating during World and European Championships is increasing, which leads to an increase of injury rates and chronic degenerative changes [5].

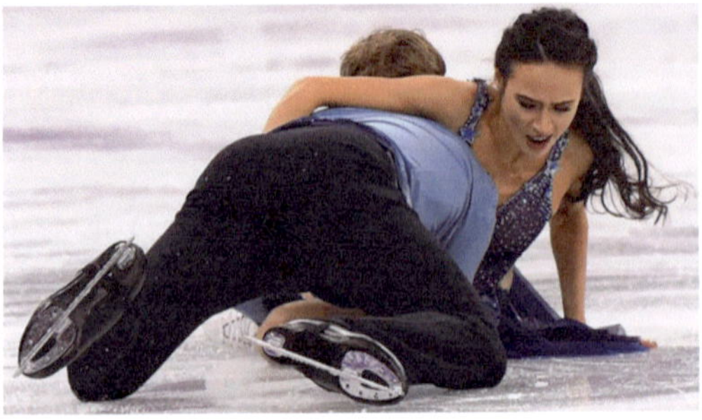

Fig. 9.1 Acute injuries predominantly occur in pair skaters

The range of figure skating injuries is wide enough—from the foot and lower-extremity injuries till the head and upper-extremity injuries [1]. It is influenced by age, gender, professional level, regularity of classes, and participation in other sports [1, 6–8]. The most common sites of injury among adolescent and adult skaters are the foot/ankle, knee, and back [1, 6]. Lower-extremity stress fractures are also quite frequent. According to Fortin, ankle injuries in medical history were reported in 27.7%, knee 18.6%, and back 15.4% [1]. In a study by Kowalczyk of adolescent figure skaters, the most common injury sites were foot/ankle with 29.3%, knee 19.0%, back 15.6%, and hip 11.7%.

Foot injuries are mostly due to overuse and include the following nosology forms: retrocalcaneal and superficial calcaneal bursitis (Fig. 9.2), toe extensor synovitis, Haglund disease, toe deformities, and corns [1, 6]. Up to half of ankle injuries are ankle sprains with less range in synchronized skating, following Achilles tendinopathy and peroneal or tibialis posterior tendinopathy [1, 6].

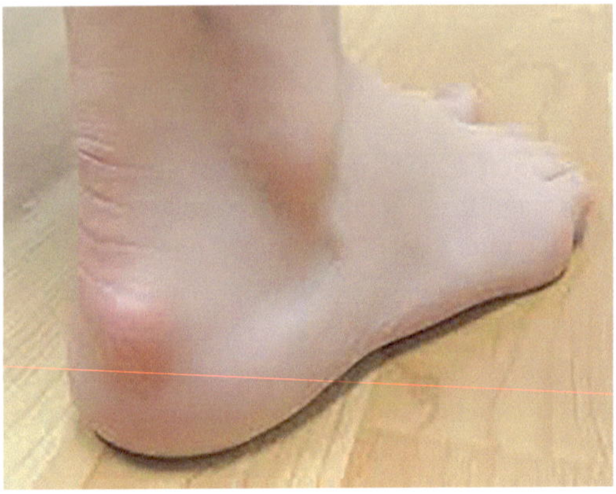

Fig. 9.2 Calcaneal bursitis is frequent in figure skating

Patellofemoral pain syndrome is widely spread among figure skaters due to the necessity of jumps and ice gliding, with the incidence of 21–32,9% [1, 6, 9]. Patellar tendonitis and Osgood-Schlatter disease are often diagnosed in young athletes. Meniscal and ligament injuries in figure skaters are rare. Lower-back pain is caused by jumps and hyperextension, torsional loads in specific movements, artistic poses (camel spin, Biellmann, etc.) with an incidence of 11–13% [10, 11]. The most common problems in lumbar spine are facet joint arthropathy, posterior column bone stress injuries, spondylolysis, and spondylolisthesis. Intervertebral disc pathology is uncommon for young athletes but increases with aging up to 63% among Olympic-level athletes [12].

Stress fractures and bone reaction typically occur in lower-extremity bones (tibia, fibula, metatarsal) (Fig. 9.3a, b) with the incidence of 11–19,8% and also in a lumbar spine with a various incidence from 4% to 45% [1, 6, 10, 11].

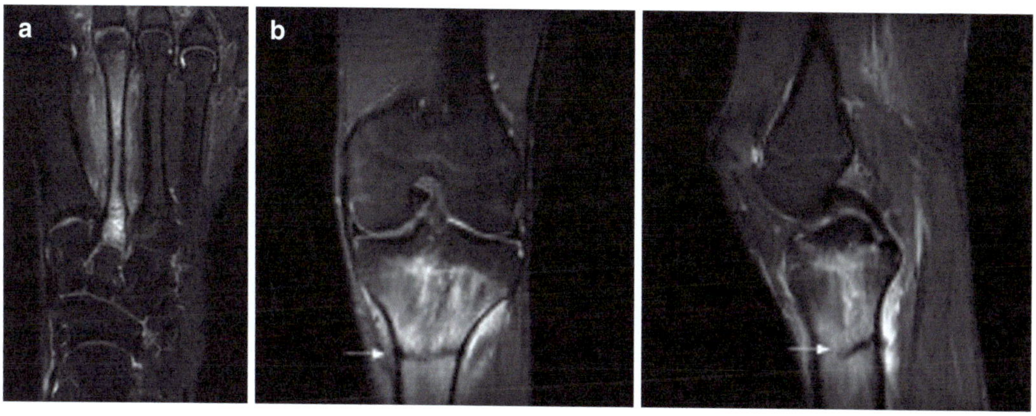

Fig. 9.3 MRI of (**a**) metatarsal and tibial (**b**) stress fractures as the most frequent stress bone injury in figure skating

9.4 Diagnosis

Diagnosis starts with anamnesis—it is necessary to understand when the pain starts, in which circumstances, and loads. During the program of scenic elements and jumps, as a result of constant cyclic loading, stress fractures can arise, especially in the lower extremities [5, 13]. In addition to the basic questions related to the occurrence of pain, it is necessary to ask in detail what kind of boots the athlete is training (new shoes or not, custom made shoes, type of lacing, usage of orthopedic insoles).

Assessment of the skin and swelling area, pain level, and function impairment should be carried out. Sport shoes play a significant role in the development of injuries—pain localization should be noted relative to the boot. Also, extremity anatomical structure and feet deformities (pes cavus or pes planus) affect the distribution of the load in different ways compared to the normal anatomy [1].

Bursitis is a typical overuse injury in figure skating and occurs more often in the area of the medial malleolus, lateral malleolus, and along the anterior surface (tibial muscle tendons due to constant pressure from the tight parts of the ridge) [13]. Tendinopathy diagnosis is based on clinical symptoms, localization of pain, and performance of specific tests depending on localization. However, in Achilles tendinopathy, pain can be localized both at the attachment point, and diffuse thickening of the tendon itself is possible [14, 15].

Imaging studies should begin with x-ray to assess the bone structure and the presence or absence of bone outgrowths and fractures. X-ray may be useful to detect Haglund disease, Osgood-Schlatter disease, and stress fractures [9]. MRI is necessary to observe bone reaction and changes in back pain and for the diagnosis of stress fractures (Fig. 9.3), inflammation of the periosteum, bursitis, achillopathy, muscle damage, tendon avulsion, and anterior knee pain [14, 16, 17].

9.5 Treatment Options

9.5.1 Foot and Ankle Injuries

Ankle sprains are probably the most common acute injuries in figure skaters. Sprains often occur during off-ice training sessions. Treatment includes ice, elevation, NSAIDs in gels locally and in tablets, reduction of sport activity, and fixation in a brace for several weeks.

Malleolar bursitis is a common injury due to continued pressure and friction of the boot at the region of the medial malleolus. This condition can develop acutely or chronically and typically responds well to conservative treatment. Above all, boot modification should be done. Adding various types of padding around the tender area helps relieve pressure points. Conservative treatment includes physical therapy aiming to reduce inflammation, ice, NSAIDs, and reduction of sport activity. In rare cases, puncturing to remove fluid and corticosteroid injection may be required (1). Surgical resection of chronically inflamed bursa can be successful but is rarely necessary. Achilles tendinopathy occurs from repetitive plantarflexion and deep dorsiflexion at the ankle during stroking. Again, firstly, boot modification is necessary to improve the fit through the heel and then training modification with reduction of hours per day and number of jumps per day. Anti-inflammatory medication and ice massage are helpful combined with physical therapy (1). The skater should be taught appropriate stretching and strengthening exercises, and gradually, a plyometric strengthening program should be developed so that the athlete has a calf suitable to perform the skating jumping maneuvers.

9.5.2 Patellofemoral Pain

The constant load on the extensors during jumping and sliding on ice increases stress on the anterior part of the knee joint. This contributes to the appearance of patellofemoral pain syndrome and Osgood-Schlatter disease and leads to tendinopathies (1). The main approach in treatment of overload injuries is load reduction, as well as limitation of provocative movements. Treatment options should include exercise therapy (strengthening, stretching, and aerobic exercise), joint mobilizations, patellofemoral taping, neuromuscular electrical stimulation, and neuromuscular training [18]. Stretching exercises for the quadriceps, hamstring, and iliotibial band may reduce the risk of anterior knee pain and decrease load to knee cap.

9.5.3 Back Injures

Since the most common problems are facet joint arthropathy, column bone stress injuries, spondylolysis, and spondylolisthesis, the treatment consists in restriction or modification of loading and physical therapy (1). Exercise program includes strengthening of core abdominal muscles, stretching of hip flexors, and anti-lordotic exercises for the lumbar spine.

9.5.4 Stress Fractures

Stress fractures and bone reaction, typically of lower-extremity bones, are usually treated conservatively. These overuse injuries usually result in working on one particular maneuver. First, load reduction with the elimination of the particular element from the practice must be performed. Sometimes, completely removing loads on the lower extremity are needed, with the use of crutches and a cast boot, until healing occurs. In rare case, surgical treatment with fixation of big segments is necessary [14, 16].

9.5.5 Hip Injuries

Due to triple and quadruple jumps, muscle strains of the hip flexors, adductor muscles, and anterior iliac crest avulsions and groin pain are commonly seen in skaters. Treatment includes rest from the offending activity and anti-inflammatories, followed by physical therapy. However, these injuries may take 2–3 months to heal [1, 19].

9.6 RTP (Return to Performance)

9.6.1 Patellofemoral Pain (Anterior Knee Pain)

The return-to-sport stage in treatment process for patients with *anterior knee pain* should involve limb functional testing (limb symmetry index LSI), progressive sport-specific drills, and gradual athlete's involvement in full training process. Isokinetic dynamometry for hip muscle strength testing, hop testing, and functional muscle testing such as single-leg squat or single-leg bridge should be performed to assess the athlete readiness to go back to sports [20].

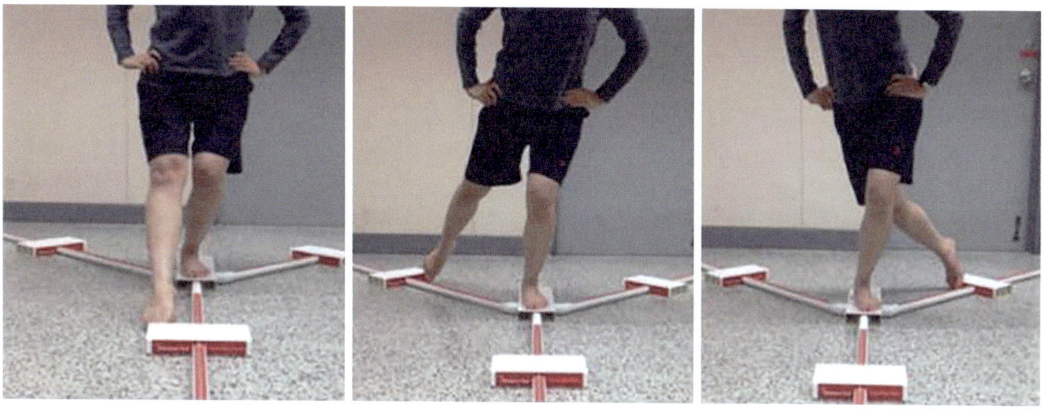

Fig. 9.4 Y-Balance test

9.6.2 Ankle Sprain

There is still lack of objective tests and criteria that could precisely predict the rate of re-injuries [21]. When analyzing criteria of RTP, all functional limitations should be restored, such as cardiovascular system endurance, no apprehension from the athlete. Although ankle sprain scores are not validated in terms of RTP, they could possibly evaluate the functional condition of the lower extremity and the effectiveness of physical therapy. Moreover, there is a list of functional tests that could be performed to analyze the functional condition of injuries leg, such as hop tests (single-hop or triple-hop tests, side-hop tests) or balance tests (Y-balance test) (Fig. 9.4).

9.6.3 Back Pain

It is still unclear what is the most objective criteria for RTP in athletes with LBP. However, the University of Queensland (Australia) estimated that return participation continuum should include full range of motion in the spine, pain-free extension, no medication use, decrease in morning stiffness, and performance confidence as a part of psychological readiness for RTP [22].

9.7 Prevention

Prevention strategies should include off-ice training focused on strengthening, stretching, and conditioning drills. The main goals are:

Neuromuscular proprioceptive and coordination drills on stable surfaces progressed with rhythmic stabilization and unstable platforms [23]
Jumping exercises (landing progressed to jumps, from triple to quadruple) [5]
Core and upper body strength exercises for compensation for forces encountered on the ice.
Modifying knee extensor mechanism (rectus femoris), including proper flexibility + quadriceps strengthening in cable in prone position to prevent patellofemoral or anterior knee pain.
Ankle joint flexibility drills (proper Achilles stretching) to keep foot dorsiflexion [5]
Calf muscle strengthening.
Unilateral exercises both strengthening and balance.

Treatment options include skating modifications, jump technique assessment, reducing the number of jumps per day, and increasing the volume of ice-time a day or a week [14].

Skating shoes should fit properly to guarantee ankle stability and mobility at the same time. Oversized skating boots may lead to subcutaneous bursitis, whereas tight boots can cause the restriction of ankle motion in the sagittal plane and development of ankle and foot non-physiological conditions and deformities as responses to stress, which can limit ankle's role in absorbing jump landing forces [5].

References

1. Han JS, Geminiani ET, Micheli LJ. Epidemiology of figure skating injuries: a review of the literature. Sports Health. 2018;10(6):532–7.
2. Yu R, Park H, Lee J. Figure skating simulation from video. Comput Graph Forum. 2019;38(7):225–34.
3. Vescovi J, VanHeest J. The science of figure skating. 1st ed. Routledge; 2018.
4. Fortin JD, Roberts D. Competitive figure skating injuries. Pain Phys. 2003;6(3):313–8.
5. Rauer T, Pape HC, Knobe M, Pohlemann T, Ganse B. Figure skating: increasing numbers of revolutions in jumps at the European and world championships. PLoS One. 2022;17(11):e0265343.
6. Kowalczyk A, Geminiani E, Dahlberg B, Micheli L, Sugimoto D. Pediatric and adolescent figure skating injuries: a 15-year retrospective review. Clin J Sport Med. 2019;
7. Sugimoto D, Jackson SS, Howell DR, Meehan WP, Stracciolini A. Association between training volume and lower extremity overuse injuries in young female athletes: implications for early sports specialization. Phys Sportsmed. 2019;47(2):199–204.
8. Sugimoto D, Lambrinakos-Raymond K, Kobelski GP, Geminiani ET, Stracciolini A, Meehan WP. Sport specialization of female figure skaters: cumulative effects on low back injuries. Phys Sportsmed. 2021;49(4):463–8.
9. Campanelli V, Piscitelli F, Verardi L, Maillard P, Sbarbati A. Lower extremity overuse conditions affecting figure skaters during daily training. Orthop J Sports Med. 2015;3(7):2325967115596517.
10. Dubravcic-Simunjak S, Pecina M, Kuipers H, Moran J, Haspl M. The incidence of injuries in elite junior figure skaters. Am J Sports Med. 2003;31(4):511–7.
11. d'Hemecourt PA, Luke A. Sport-specific biomechanics of spinal injuries in aesthetic athletes (dancers, gymnasts, and figure skaters). Clin Sports Med. 2012;31(3):397–408.
12. Goldstein JD, Berger PE, Windler GE, Jackson DW. Spine injuries in gymnasts and swimmers. An epidemiologic investigation. Am J Sports Med. 1991;19(5):463–8.
13. Fröhlich S, Zimmermann SM, Sutter R, Frey WO, Spörri J. Medial malleolar bursitis in an elite competitive alpine skier: a case report. Curr Sports Med Rep. 2020;19(10):399–401.
14. Bradley MA. Prevention and treatment of foot and ankle injuries in figure skaters. Curr Sports Med Rep. 2006;5(5):258–61.
15. Leikin JB. Foreword for: current understanding of the diagnosis and management of the tendinopathy: an update from the lab to the clinical practice. Dis Mon. 2022;68(10):101313.
16. Ryazantsev MS, Zaripov AR, Afanasyev AP, Maysigov MN, Magnitskaya NE, Ilyin DO. Long-term results of medical treatment for lower extremity stress fractures. Nauchno-prakticheskaia revmatologiia. 2020;58(1):102–5.
17. Webb B, Kenning JH, Guzman A, Slater L, Mangum LC. Lumbopelvic-hip complex contribution during lower extremity screening tests in elite figure skaters. J Athl Train. 2021;18
18. Capin JJ, Snyder-Mackler L. The current management of patients with patellofemoral pain from the physical therapist's perspective. Ann Jt. 2018;3:40.
19. Porter EB, Young CC, Niedfeldt MW, Gottschlich LM. Sport-specific injuries and medical problems of figure skaters. WMJ. 2007;106(6):330–4.
20. Theisen BJ, Larson PD, Chambers CC. Optimizing rehabilitation and return to sport in athletes with anterior knee pain using a biomechanical perspective. Arthrosc Sports Med Rehabil. 2022;4(1):e199–207.
21. D'Hooghe P, Cruz F, Alkhelaifi K. Return to play after a lateral ligament ankle sprain. Curr Rev Musculoskelet Med. 2020;13(3):281–8.
22. Ardern CL, Glasgow P, Schneiders A, Witvrouw E, Clarsen B, Cools A. Consensus statement on return to sport from the first world congress in sports physical therapy, Bern. Br J Sports Med. 2016;50(14):853–64.
23. Vuurberg G, Hoorntje A, Wink LM, van der Doelen BFW, van den Bekerom MP, Dekker R. Diagnosis, treatment and prevention of ankle sprains: update of an evidence-based clinical guideline. Br J Sports Med. 2018;52(15):956.

10 Pole Dance

Henrique Jones and Susana Pialgata

10.1 Introduction

10.1.1 History

Despite its controversial origins and stigma surrounding it, pole dancing has become more widely accepted and celebrated as a form of art and athleticism. Pole dance, as we know it today, is quite a young and developing sport and art. But it has great potential. And to understand this, you need to learn more about the *history of pole dance*. In the twelfth century, Mallakhamb, a sport born in India, combines acrobatics and yoga elements on a pole 35–55 cm in diameter (the pole narrowed in height) [1]. The word "Malla" means "wrestler," and "Khamb" means "pole" or "column." The earliest mention of Mallakhamb is in the Indian classical *Manasollasa*, written in AD 1135. The emergence of the Chinese pole sport is also associated with the twelfth century. That's when men in China started using rubber-coated poles 5–9 meters high to perform acrobatic tricks. Traditionally, again, it is mostly a man's sport, existing, and is still popular today. In Europe, Maypole dancing is a pagan dance of fertility during which girls danced around the May tree (any high tree or pillar) decorated with flowers. In a sense, the ancestor of the pole dance can also be called tribal ritual dances in Africa. During these rituals, engaged women danced around a high pillar, showing how she wanted her future husband to make love to her [1].

H. Jones (✉) · S. Pialgata
Hospital da Luz, Setúbal Orthopedic Surgery and Sports Medicine, Montijo Orthopedic Sports Med Clinic, Setubal, Portugal

10.1.2 Characteristics of the Sport/ Art

Over the past years, pole dancing has become widely known. Sometimes, it is combined with other choreographies or acrobatic moves. Quite frequently, dancing shows are held in dancing schools along with competitions and even circus shows where the origins of pole dancing can be found. Whether being a man or a woman, an amateur or professional dancer, learning skills and competition are gradually increasing, and therefore, standards become higher. There is no age limit on pole dancing, and there's really nothing that a child couldn't physically do that an adult can do *on a dance pole*. There are some children who might want to take classes with adults initially so they have someone serving as a role model. The reasons why kids might want to do pole dances are just as diverse as the adult reasons. Kids are just as capable of learning pole tricks if their bodies are developed enough. There's really no minimum age requirement to start doing tricks at all. Not everyone is able to stick "inversions," but inversions are not required

H. Jones, A. Lukaszenko (eds.), *Injury Prevention and Care in Artistic Sports*,
https://doi.org/10.1007/978-3-032-18105-3_10

for anyone to be successful in pole fitness classes at the beginning. Many young pole dancers start out with traditional *basic beginners' moves and tricks* as a "bird" and "basic plank." As they develop more strength, children are able to learn moves that are traditionally seen in adult classes, but at their own pace. Besides being a sport, it is also a very beautiful kind of dance. Many elements are performed gracefully and plastically, which requires certain dancing skills from the performer.

Pole dancing can be consider an art but also a sport with specific learning course, technical skills, adapted movements, training, and competition. Like other kinds of exercise, *injuries* may also occur in pole dancing, which are relevant to *the kind of exercise, technique, and physical condition*. This is the reason why competent coaching and prevention should be the rule in its practice with important ground prevention exercises (Fig. 10.1).

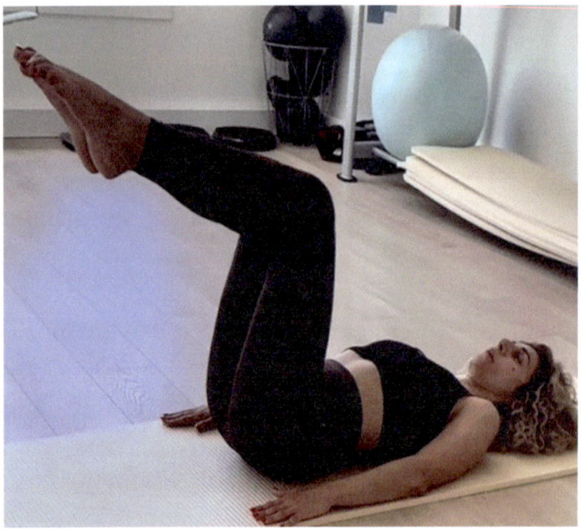

Fig. 10.1 Prevention exercises on the floor are important to prevent pole injuries

10.2 Specificities of the Sport/Art

Pole dancing requires aerobic and aerial skillfulness, flexibility of the joints, and elasticity in the soft parts of the body (muscles, tendons, ligaments, etc.) especially of the lower limbs and the trunk, while the requirements of the exercises are extremely intense. Pole dancing is a combination of various disciplines, including acrobatics, sport gymnastic, and dance. Developing this skill is associated with an increased risk for locomotor system injuries, which are inherent in amateur and professional pole dance trainings.

The kinds of exercises are usually prolonged, mostly in the upper limbs and the trunk. This means that the muscles must be fully coordinated and immediately respond in any case (Fig. 10.2). The athlete, on his behalf, must have full concentration and full understanding of his body position toward the pole and the ground. She, or he, should perceive external stimuli, such as gravity and the direction of the pole. All these must be taken into consideration by the trainee because he is not used to them in his everyday life.

10.2.1 Aerial Pole Dance

Originating as a unique extension of pole dancing and aerial arts, this form incorporates a suspended pole that moves and rotates, allowing dancers to soar through the air. Unlike stationary poles, flying poles require specific strength, flexibility, and coordination to perform adequate acrobatic maneuvers (Fig. 10.2).

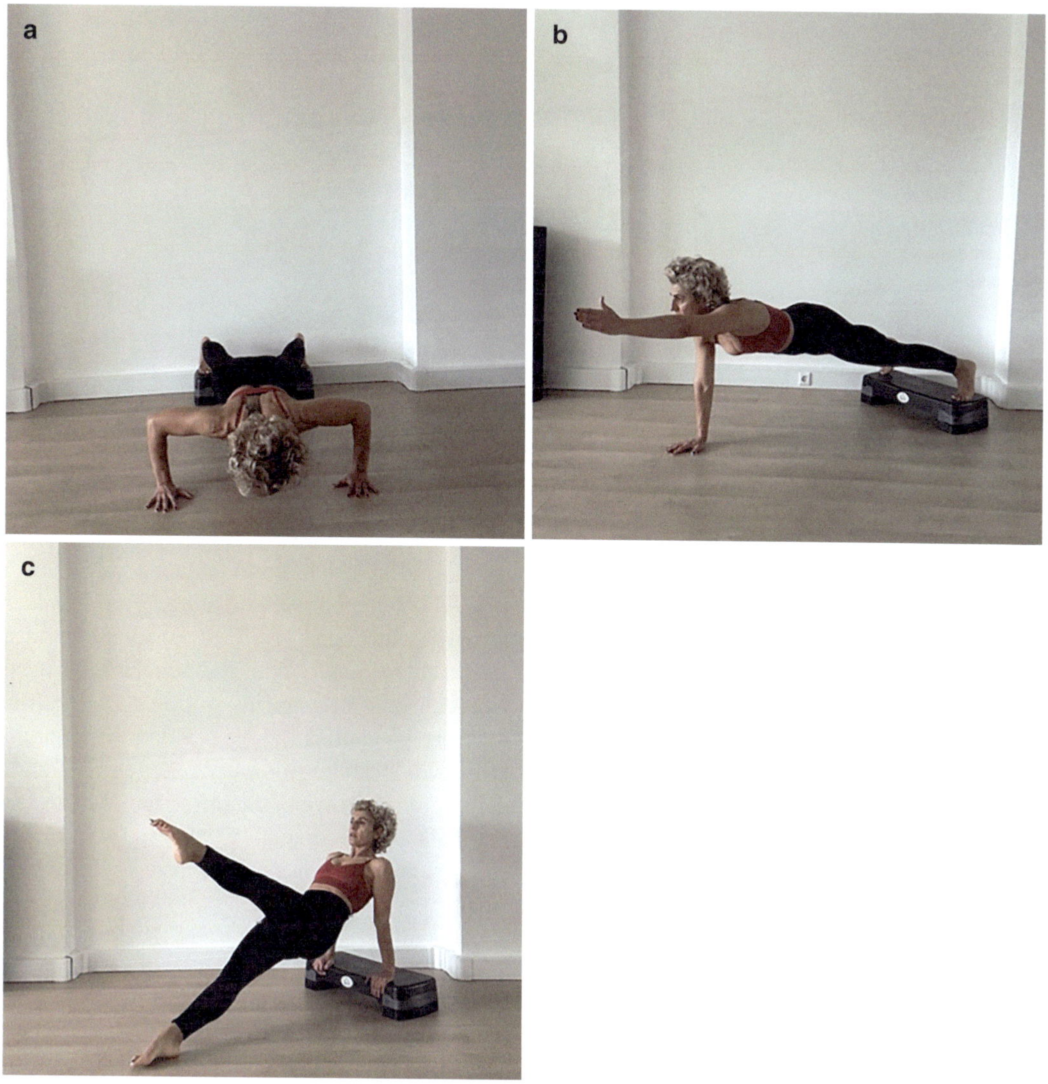

Fig. 10.2 (**a–c**) Coordination and strength for pole dance preparation

10.3 Epidemiology of More Frequent Injuries

Injuries in pole dancing vary from burns and bruises to even more serious conditions, which might torment the athlete for a long time. However, the most common type of injury is bruising generated due to friction and pressure between the athlete's skin (usually forearm and leg) and the pole, and generally it is not a serious injury (Fig. 10.3a, b).

Other injuries are caused by overuse of the upper limbs; muscle spasms in the neck, chest, and lumbar area; and muscle ruptures in the lower limbs.

Between those injuries, we can stand out tendinosis in rotator cuff; sprains and strains in the wrist, forearm, and intercostal associated with other injuries like carpal tunnel syndrome; trigger point and intense muscle spasms in the trapezoid, deltoid, rhomboid, and elevator of the scapula (shoulder blade); as well as hamstring injuries.

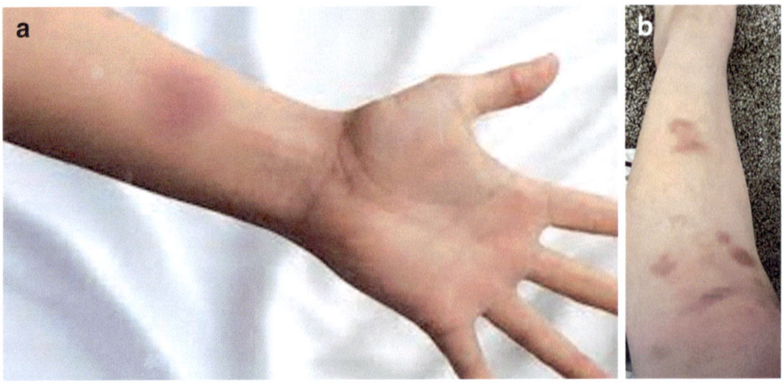

Fig. 10.3 Pole dancing habitual bruising injuries

Rotator cuff injuries are one of the most common in pole dancing, and that's because they can be caused by micro-trauma to the muscles over weeks, months, or even years beforehand. Micro-trauma can be caused by hanging your body weight from your shoulder during pole classes without engaging your muscles correctly. Finally, injuries caused by falls can vary from simple fractures, usually in the upper limbs, shoulder, and elbow dislocation, and (rarely) head and brain injuries.

According to Mariusz Naczk et al. in 2020, [2] pole dancing had many positive physiological effects, but pole dancers should be aware that pole dancing and behavior associated with training significantly increased the risk of injury. Results of their study indicate that many attempts at weight loss are connected with high risk of acute injury. They also concluded that pole dancers possessed significantly greater muscle strength and lower back and hamstring muscle flexibility compared to untrained controls. Pole dancers had significantly less body fat and significantly more muscle mass in the upper limbs compared to untrained controls. During 2 years of pole dance training, 36.7% of the dancers had sustained acute injuries (mainly muscle, shoulder joint, and wrist injuries), and 80% of the dancers had sustained a chronic injury. Most injuries occurred during handsprings, twines, and carousel performances. Moreover, pole dancers experienced more menstrual irregularities than the controls.

The work of Nicholas J. et al. in 2022 [9] reported a total of 103 injuries occurred, 62.1% of which were sudden onset and 37.9% gradual onset. Mechanism of onset included 54.4% acute and 45.6% repetitive in nature. The shoulder (20.4%) and thigh (11.7%, majority hamstring) were the most reported anatomic injury sites. Non-contact mechanisms accounted for the majority of injuries (57.3%). The most reported primary contributor to injury onset at the shoulder were maneuvers characterized by loaded internal humeral rotation (33.3%) and at the hamstring were maneuvers and postures involving front splits (100%).

Also in Lee, JY et al.'s study (2020) [4], most commonly reported injuries were shoulder-related (54.5%) injuries and wrist (34.2%) and back (24.7%) injuries. 75.5% of injuries were acutely sustained. Pole dancers who were 40 and above were 3.7 times more likely to need more than 3 months to recover from their pole injuries than those who were aged from 19 to 29 years. Participants with 3–6 years of pole sport experience were at 3.9 times higher risk for moderate/severe injuries than those who had less experience.

10.4 Diagnosis and Treatment Options

Diagnosis of mild pole injuries are clinical, and topical treatment is normally enough. More severe overuse or traumatic injuries must be confirmed with x-ray, sonography, or MRI. Some topical applications have interesting therapeutic results: ice pack or a cold compress early on to minimize damage for a period of 15 min each area for 2 h. Some products like arnica gel (anti-inflammatory properties that may help reduce pain, swelling, and bruises), aloe vera (cooling, anti-inflammatory effect and vascular repair), and Vitamin C and K (tissue repair) are also suggested.

Muscle injuries [3] represent one of the most common traumas in sports medicine. They have different clinical manifestations depending on the trauma mechanism: laceration, contusion, and strain. The range of lesions vary from minor partial ruptures to complete ruptures of the muscle. The muscular tissue has a capacity to regenerate, and the healing process consists of regeneration of muscle fibers and formation of a connective tissue scar. The healing is also greatly dependent on the ingrowth of vascularity and regeneration of intramuscular nerve branches.

10.5 RTP (Return to Performance)

Once pain has subsided, exercises to strengthen the shoulder can help toward a full recovery, and you should have total rest from pole dancing until the area is free from discomfort. Recovery time can vary from 3 to 6 weeks but often recurs if no strengthening of the muscle is done to prevent a repeat injury. In muscle injuries, the decision regarding the appropriate timing of the return to sports-specific training can be based on two simple and inexpensive measures: [3, 4] the ability to stretch the injured muscle as much as the healthy contralateral muscle and [6] the pain-free use of the injured muscle in basic movements. When the athlete states that she/he has reached this point in recovery, then permission to gradually start sports-specific training is granted.

Pole dancers with lower level of experience in training, who sustained an injury, and who had a shorter pause between the moment of injury and the return to performance, and thus who did not fully recover, have higher odds of sustaining a re-injury. Sport-specific injury prevention strategies should be developed and implemented in this cohort, since over 85% of pole dancers reported sustaining some kind of injury [4, 5].

10.6 Prevention

Most sports have a common pattern of injury, either by repetitive overuse of muscles, by muscle imbalance, or from some sort of repetitive strain. In the discipline of Pole dance practitioners must have a systematic discipline of moves to keep bodies proper response to exercise and, training both sides, is important to prevent muscle imbalances [6]. The most important factors that can protect pole dancers by acute injuries are a well-performed warm-up and balanced diet [7, 8].

When on the pole be sure that you wear the appropriate clothes. Having loose clothing can cause slip and slide on the pole and generate bruises. If wearing tight-fitting pole dancing clothes, the chance of getting bruises decreases. Sticky pole wear will also help you with grip and pressure. Specific designed fabric for pole dancing means avoiding hard grip to maintain friction on the pole. Having the correct pole wear will let you perform much better and help avoid injury.

The work of Nicholas J. et al. [9] shows that pole dancers are at a high risk for injuries. Future research is needed to understand the biomechanical demand of maneuvers and training characteristics of pole dancing (e.g., workload and recovery) to guide the development of preventative interventions, particularly targeted toward the shoulder and hamstring.

References

1. History of Pole Dance: from 12 century Mallahamba to today, January 29, 2020 by Emma Bolton https://dancebibles.com/history-of-pole-dance/
2. Naczk M, Kowalewska A, Naczk A. The risk of injuries and physiological benefits of pole dancing. J Sports Med Phys Fitness. 2020;60(6):883–8. https://doi.org/10.23736/S0022-4707.20.10379-7.
3. Lehto MU, Järvinen MJ. Muscle injuries, their healing process and treatment. Ann Chir Gynaecol. 1991;80(2):102–8.

4. Lee JY, Lin L, Tan A. Prevalence of pole dance injuries from a global online survey. J Sports Med Phys Fitness. 2020;60(2):270–5. https://doi.org/10.23736/S0022-4707.19.09957-2.
5. Best TM, Hunter KD. Muscle injury and repair. Phys Med Rehabil Clin N Am. 2000;11(2):251–66.
6. Markert CD, Merrick MA, Kirby TE, Devor ST. Nonthermal ultrasound and exercise in skeletal muscle regeneration. Arch Phys Med Rehabil. 2005;86(7):1304–10.
7. Gołuchowska AM, Humka MI. Types of the locomotor system injuries and frequency of occurrence in women pole dancers. J Sports Med Phys Fitness. 2022;62(5):661–6. https://doi.org/10.23736/S0022-4707.21.12239-X.
8. Szopa A, Domagalska-Szopa M, Urbańska A, Grygorowicz M. Factors associated with injury and re-injury occurrence in female pole dancers. Sci Rep. 2022;12(1):33. https://doi.org/10.1038/s41598-021-04000-5.
9. Nicholas J, Weir G, Alderson JA, Stubbe JH, van Rijn RM, Dimmock JA, Jackson B, Donnelly CJ. Incidence, mechanisms, and characteristics of injuries in pole dancers: a prospective cohort study. Med Probl Perform. 2022;37(3):151–64. https://doi.org/10.21091/mppa.2022.3022.

Rhythmic Gymnastics

11

Natalie Brettler

Rhythmic gymnastics (RG) is a sport that combines artistic expression with physical performance—a combination of art and sport. The sport has evolved over time, and it is now popular worldwide with competitions held at national and international levels.

11.1 Introduction

Rhythmic gymnastics is a discipline that requires the gymnast to combine elements of dance, acrobatics, ballet, and gymnastics, performed to music, with the use of hand-held apparatuses such as ribbon, hoop, ball, clubs, and rope. This unique combination places the sport among the most demanding sports, requiring an unprecedented degree of synchronization and coordination (Fig. 11.1).

However, as with any sport, rhythmic gymnastics is not without its risks. Gymnasts are susceptible to a variety of injuries that can affect their performance and overall health. This chapter provides an overview of the history of rhythmic gymnastics, main characteristics, common injuries associated with the sport, suggested ways to prevent them, and highlights for rehabilitation.

These days, the sport is designed for women, mostly between the ages of 4 and early 20 s. There are countries around the world where men have begun practicing the sport as well; however, they are still not permitted to participate in official international competitions. Rhythmic gymnastics is comprised of two categories—individual and team. In the individual category, the gymnast

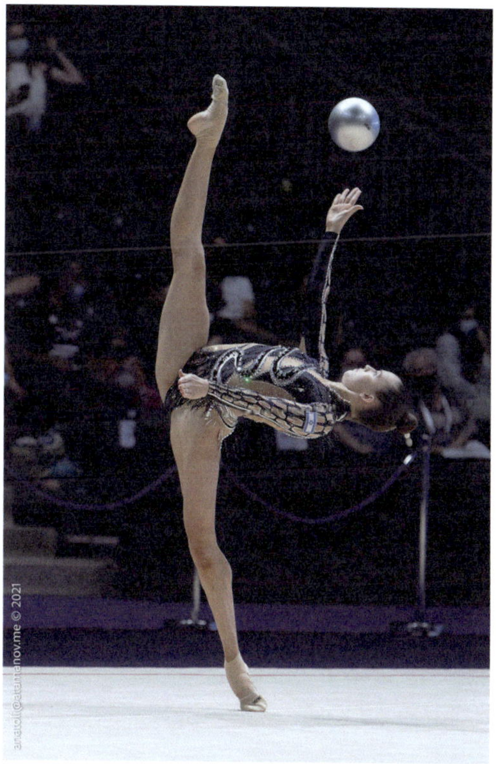

Fig. 11.1 Rhythmic gymnastics means synchronization and coordination. © Photograph by "Anatoli Atamanov". All rights reserved. Reproduced with permissions

N. Brettler (✉)
Ayelet Chen, Herzeliya, Israel

H. Jones, A. Lukaszenko (eds.), *Injury Prevention and Care in Artistic Sports*,
https://doi.org/10.1007/978-3-032-18105-3_11

performs a one-and-a-half-minute exercise alone on the floor, whereas in the team category, five gymnasts perform together using five apparatus over a period of 2.5 min.

At a competitive level over the age of 12, an individual gymnast performs with four different apparatus (drawn out of the five existing ones every 4 years). Gymnasts in the team category compete in two exercises: one with five identical apparatus and another with two combined apparatus.

Each year, at the start of the season, new exercises are built to match the music played during the exercise to its choreography and to the gymnast's leotard. The exercises are built using a strict set of rules, requiring certain elements to be performed and setting the score for the completion of each element.

Each practice session comprises of ballet, warmup, stretching, apparatus preparation, the practice of body elements, each gymnast's exercises with music, and finally fitness. The aspiration for flawless performance and a perfect combination of the different elements the sport demands—body elements requiring strength, flexibility, and speed along with swift and precise apparatus work, all to the sound of music and intricate choreography—makes the sport one of the most demanding fields in terms of practice hours, reaching up to 8–12 h a day, 6 days a week.

Most injuries will accordingly feature characteristics of overuse. The sport is characterized by the aspiration for high aesthetics. Therefore, gymnasts must maintain a low body weight. Although the sport does not feature weight categories (e.g., in Judo), gymnasts are expected to be thin and of a narrow physique.

11.2 History of Rhythmic Gymnastics

Gymnastics has a long and rich history; it is believed to have originated for the first time in Egypt as a means of entertainment for the pharaohs as early as 5000 BC. Also in ancient Greece, athletes would perform gymnastic routines to music. Rhythmic gymnastics was mainly developed in eastern Europe, In 1961, the International Gymnastics Federation (FIG) officially recognized rhythmic gymnastics as a sport. The sport's first World Championships were held in 1963, won by Soviet gymnast Ludmila Savinkova. It slowly gained popularity around the world. The sport made its Olympic debut in 1984 in Los Angeles, with Individual All-Around where Canadian Laurie Fung became the first Olympic champion in modern gymnastics. Team competitions were introduced in 1996 during Atlanta Oliympic Games.

11.3 Specific Characteristics of Rhythmic Gymnastics

There are several key characteristics of the field and of the gymnasts participating in it, which contribute to the occurrence of specific kinds of injuries.

Rhythmic gymnastics combines ballet, acrobatics, dance, and complete control over handheld apparatus. The combination of all of these demands coordination and precision, which require many hours of practice, more than in any other sport. For national competitions, it is customary to practice 6 days a week, 4–8 h a day, while gymnasts competing at the international level often reach 6 days of practice a week, 10–12 h a day. Gymnasts tend to begin practicing at an incredibly young age (around the age of four). The abundance of practice hours and the lack of ability of the body to recover commonly cause overuse injuries, typical of this sport. This phenomenon increases in tendency mostly during competitive seasons (between March and September), when we usually observe a rapid increase in training loads, and insufficient recovery could create an even greater imbalance between load and recovery and might expose gymnasts to maladaptation and higher injury risk.

One of the difficulties in the field is the lack of time to recover from an injury. Gymnasts often finish their careers at an early age—the retirement age at the international level is no higher than the early 20 s, and very few gymnasts continue to compete past it. The short career and the inability to disable the body over extended periods tend to prevent gymnasts from fully recovering from injuries or to push them into participating in competitions and practice with chronic injuries—thus causing deterioration or recurring injuries.

The aesthetics in this field matter greatly, and there is extreme meticulousness regarding the appearance of the gymnast on the floor. This includes the leotard worn by the gymnast, the meticulous hairdo, and naturally her physique as well. Gymnasts are required to conform to standards of low body weight (below 18.5 BMI) and low fat percentage (5–12% in elite gymnasts). It is therefore unsurprising to have been discovered that the incidence of eating disorders is high in athletes participating in aesthetic-type sports such as rhythmic gymnastics and gymnastics. Additionally, in most gymnasts, we can detect dysmenorrhea, which is known to be associated with an increased risk of injury (such as bone stress). The female athlete triad (disordered eating, dysmenorrhea, and osteoporosis) could be also recognized in rhythmic gymnasts. The need to keep a low body weight, along with the lack of knowledge about a balanced diet and the extended practice periods, often creates low energy availability and nutritional deficiencies that may contribute to the occurrence of injuries and make it difficult to recover from them.

Over the years, we see a significant increase in the difficulty of exercises and the abilities that gymnasts are expected to maintain. The number of elements they are required to perform in an exercise (over the same period of a minute and a half) has almost quadrupled in recent years! Furthermore, every 4 years, after the Olympics, the rules are changed by the Federation International de Gymnastique (FIG)—the score for completion of different elements changes—and the difficulty level rises throughout all categories. Those changes affect the types of injuries we see. For example, after the 2000 Sydney Olympics, the sport started incorporating many balance elements performed by balancing on one knee and by jumping from a standing position to landing directly on the knees. Such elements granted the gymnast high scores, and many gymnasts started to perform them. Naturally, elements of this type caused plenty of knee-related injuries, and so they were removed from the rules 4 years later, after the 2004 Athens Olympics. In the current set of rules, an intricate and agile apparatus performance is required, and the number of apparatus elements is unlimited. Thus, gymnasts must traverse across the floor at much higher speeds, and we observe more stress fractures in the feet. Moreover, in this ruleset, higher scores are given for elements incorporating back hyperextension—causing us to observe more back pains and stress fractures. It is probable that the frequency of different injuries will change after the Paris Olympics in 2024, along with the ruleset.

Gymnasts perform practically barefoot, only wearing specially designed gymnast toe shoes (Fig. 11.2) made of thin leather or fabric covering the toes, held by rubber bands around the heel. The sole purpose of this slipper is to reduce the friction between the foot and the surface and allow the gymnast to perform a large number of spins on one foot (part of the basic elements required in any exercise). These toe shoes do not offer support for the foot bones or the ankle.

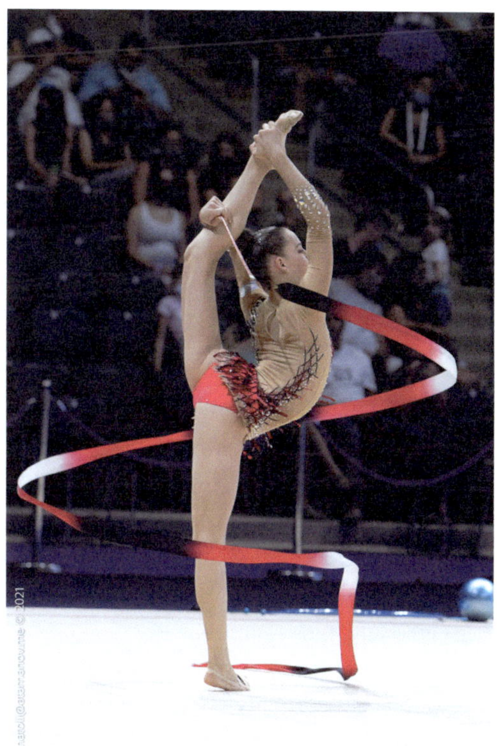

Fig. 11.2 A rhythmic gymnast performing a high-flexibility pivot while coordinating ribbon apparatus work, demonstrating the combined demands of spinal flexibility, balance, and apparatus control." © Photograph by "Anatoli Atamanov". All rights reserved. Reproduced with permissions

Much like ballet, many of the base elements of rhythmic gymnastics are performed in a split position. The gymnast has a dominant foot, which will be the front foot of the split, the other being the back foot. This applies to all split positions; standing, sitting down, lying down, and also during leaps and spins. This creates a significant imbalance between the two sides of the body, due to the dominant foot always being held in front or to the side while the other foot is always held behind.

Understanding this key characteristic of asymmetry can help with understanding the sport's overuse injuries, muscle strength imbalance, and the development of scoliosis in the back. Remembering this principle is beneficial for recovery and for building a daily fitness routine suited for the gymnast's needs.

Rhythmic gymnastics incorporates many elements requiring extreme flexibility not found in other sports. For all base elements—jumps, balance, and spins—the requirement is to reach a minimum 180-degree opening between the legs. The sport sees many participants born with hypermobility, aside from that which is developed through training.

The flexibility demanded in the field is apparent in the following joints:

Feet—The more arch apparent in the foot, and the better the pointed position, the more professional the gymnast is considered. Gymnasts dedicate a lot of practice time to stretching the foot arch, making it rounder.

Knees—Knee hyperextension is another feature that receives great attention in the field. The knees are stretched from an early age to create hyperextension. In competitions, a gymnast who fails to extend the knee further than 180 degrees will lose points for the element. As mentioned earlier, every gymnast has a dominant leg, and normally the non-dominant leg will have greater knee hyperextension because the gymnast will lean on it in elements of balance necessary in any exercise.

Thighs—One of the known characteristics of the sport is flexibility elements performed by gymnasts. The requirement is to extend over 180 degrees between the legs in a split. To reach such flexibility, gymnasts spend at least an hour stretching in every practice session (and oftentimes more than that). The stretches are static and dynamic. To complete an over-180-degree split, gymnasts practice by sitting in a split position with one leg laid on a ladder. The more flexible the gymnast becomes, the higher she will be able to put her leg up the ladder. Sometimes, coaches tend to passively stretch gymnasts—such extreme flexes could cause thigh labral tears and thigh pains highly common among gymnasts.

Back—Many elements require extreme back flexibility, some of them only being counted if the head touches the back foot or the buttock. Some gymnasts reach the sport with hypermobility in the back or in the legs. They all stretch daily in order to increase back flexibility. At times, during the performance of elements requiring increased back mobility, engagement of the abdomen is disregarded, and gymnasts perform the exercise without sufficient stability in the back and abdominal area, causing back pain and stress fractures.

Shoulders—High mobility in the shoulder girdle is also required in gymnastics. The back is expected to be straight, the chest open, and the shoulders protracted. Thus, shoulder girdle mobility is highly regarded—some gymnasts are able to move their arms, with their hands held together, backward over the head and all the way to the buttock without separating their hands from one another.

Shortening of the muscles in the posterior compartment of the leg (Gastrocnemius, Soleus, and Plantaris): With gymnasts spending many practice hours standing in a *relevé* position, most of them experience a shortening of those muscles, which contributes to the formation of medial collapse in the feet (pes planus), along with all associated consequences.

Medial collapse of the foot (pes planus) is usually accompanied by a medial collapse in the knee (knee valgus or valgus collapse). Perhaps one of the most surprising phenomena is the pes planus observed in a notable percentage of gymnasts. There are several contributing factors to it—shortening of the gastrocnemius and soleus muscles as mentioned above, weakness in muscles performing an inversion of the foot, mainly the tibialis anterior and tibialis posterior and external rotation of the hip. The medial collapse in the foot will usually also create a valgus collapse in any action of a close kinematic chain. Those might generate wrong techniques, pains, and injuries like those detailed in the chapter about common injuries in the sport.

11.4 Type of Injuries, Treatment, and Prevention in Rhythmic Gymnastics

Despite the beauty and grace of rhythmic gymnastics, the sport can be physically demanding and stressful on the body. The combination of all the unique catachrestic of the sport that were mentioned in the chapter above are all potential risk factors for overuse injuries; not surprisingly, the most common injuries in rhythmic gymnastics are overuse injuries to the back, hips, knees, and feet. The ankles are especially vulnerable to acute injuries.

Most injuries in rhythmic gymnastics are not severe, but rather challenging in terms of the short recovery time. As opposed to other fields where retirement ages are higher, at a competitive level, it is impossible to disable the gymnast for extensive time periods with no practice. A hiatus longer than a month or two will make it highly difficult for the gymnast to return to competitive form. This is why my motto is: "Do everything that's possible, except for what's impossible." It means that if the gymnast has a stress fracture in the foot and cannot perform a standing exercise, she can instead be given fitness/stretching/apparatus exercises to perform sitting or lying down. She can also be given the exercise to be performed without carrying additional weight—i.e., split jumps while hanging on a ladder (with no additional weight). This principle allows her to maintain overall fitness and strengthen different areas until she is able to perform the standing exercise. Working in this method reduces the "return to perform" time after an injury or at times when load reduction is needed.

Below are some of the most common injuries associated with rhythmic gymnastics by body parts, characteristics of the injury, contributing factors, and suggestions for preventing these injuries.

11.4.1 Foot Injuries

One of the most common injuries in the field is overuse injury—stress fractures in the feet. Gymnasts practice barefoot with only gymnast toe shoes made of thin fabric covering the front part of the foot. Due to the prolonged practice sessions and time spent standing on tiptoes (*relevé*), many gymnasts suffer from stress fractures in the feet, mostly around the second and third metatarsus area—where most of the body weight rests while standing on tiptoes. The daily load, combined with the lack of vitamin D, inadequate diet, amenorrhea, insufficient sleep, stress, and insufficient time for the body to recover between practice sessions, contributes to the formation of stress fractures in gymnasts' feet. This is often a recurring injury, and gymnasts who used to suffer from stress fractures tend to develop pain when the load increases. The gymnast will feel pain under any weight (walking, *relevé* standing, jumps, and any form of standing on foot). In physical examination, we will observe tenderness to palpation or percussion, and therefore bony tenderness should elicit further imaging to determine the presence of a stress reaction or stress fracture.

11.5 Prevention

Due to stress fractures being caused by several contributing factors, a substantial part of preventing them will consist of paying extra care to those factors, such as focused strengthening of foot and ankle muscles, getting sufficient sleep (at least 8 h a night), periodical blood tests to detect deficiencies, and adequate diet.

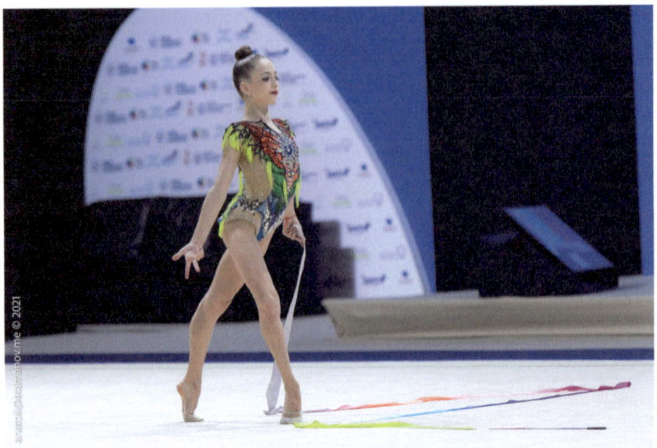

Fig. 11.3 The aesthetics in rhythmic gymnastics matter greatly." © Photograph by "Anatoli Atamanov". All rights reserved. Reproduced with permissions

Moreover, when signs of overuse or stress fractures appear, it is recommended to reduce weight carrying for a period of at least 3 weeks or a month. When the fracture heals, the gymnast will no longer feel any pain while carrying weight.

11.5.1 Notes for Rehabilitation

If the case is that of overuse, weight carrying can be omitted from most areas of training: ballet, warmup, and fitness can be performed sitting or lying down. The gymnast will be instructed not to perform any jumps or relevé/one-foot elements at all. At times when carrying weight is necessary, the gymnast should wear training shoes to protect the foot as much as possible. This way the gymnast can practice apparatus work, flexibility, and strength while at the same time allowing the foot to recover.

If stress fractures are detected (through clinical examination and x-ray or CT), the instruction is then to omit any action requiring weight carrying on the feet for a minimum of 3 weeks (the exact time depending on the severity of the fracture). All other components of the training can be performed sitting or lying down. During the entire period of weight removal, it is important to pay attention to strengthening the ankle, knee, thigh, and core muscles. Proprioceptive training of the feet can be performed lying down. The time until full return to performance will be determined usually by clinical indicators—the gymnast should report that she does not feel any pain during weight carrying. The return to performance should be gradual and very attentive to the gymnast's sensations. In addition to weight removal, the conservative treatment will naturally include physiotherapy treatment. Furthermore, there is scientific evidence on the positive effect of a Low-Intensity Pulsed Ultrasound (LIPUS Fig. 11.3) device for stimulation of bone healing, which suggests a positive effect of LIPUS in nonunion fractures with healing rates of around 85%.

11.6 Hallux Valgus

Hallux valgus is defined as a progressive abnormality in the degree of lateral deviation of the big toe at the metatarsophalangeal (MTP) joint, resulting in the formation of a bony bump on the side of the foot and may involve pain at the medial aspect of the first metatarsal head [4]. This condition has been reported to be more prevalent in female athletes (Fig. 11.4), especially in those who participate in sports that require repeated standing on *relevé*—a movement in which the gymnast rises on tips of toes. The gymnast must place their center of mass on top of the *relevé* and mainly on the first metatarsophalangeal joint. The repetitive microtrauma and excessive pressure on the first metatarsophalangeal joint during training and competition are thought

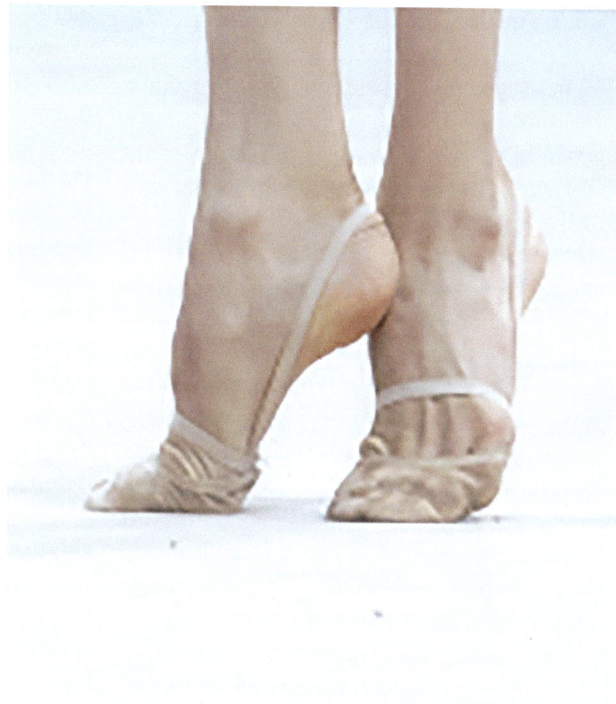

Fig. 11.4 Hallux valgus seems to be more prevalent in female athletes

to play a significant role in the development of this condition together with genetic factors and foot structure. Accordingly, it was reported that rhythmic gymnasts' hallux angles are significantly greater than those of corresponding age matched students, and with the prevalence of the deformity, their hallux angle was larger than 20°, increased 4.7 times more than that of the non-athlete students [1].

11.6.1 Prevention

Non-operative methods for prevention include wearing an orthosis and engaging in specific exercises. The effectiveness of orthosis is subject to conjecture and problematic for rhythmic gymnasts to wear during practice. Exercises of abduction and flexion of the big toe—showed to reduce the hallux valgus angle and hallux valgus angle during active abduction and increase the cross-sectional area of the abductor hallucis muscle [3]. This specific exercise can also be used for prevention and during the early stages of hallux valgus (HV), to prevent further increases in the HV angle [2].

Along with this exercise, it can be beneficial to release the abductor hallucis muscle by self-release with a small ball or foam roller or by a physical therapist and stretch the muscles and fascia of the plantar part of the foot and the posterior and medial compartment of the calf muscles.

11.6.2 Notes for Rehabilitation

All methods suggested above for prevention are also applicable for treatment, due to the treatment being conservative and not surgical for most gymnasts—this is due to the recovery time from surgery being very long, and any surgical outcome short of perfect can result in a serious blow to the gymnast's career. In addition to everything mentioned above, during practices and competitions, a small, elastic separation between the toes can be self-made using tapes, which can be used for practicing in toe shoes and does not interfere with the movement of the foot.

11.6.3 Ankle Injuries

The most common acute injury in rhythmic gymnastics is ankle sprains. Sprains have been reported to range from 11% to 50%, depending on the study population across all levels and ages [5, 13].

Gymnasts practice barefoot and perform jumps and swift movements on the floor while holding a handheld apparatus, with their eyes mostly set on the instrument. The practice sessions are held for many hours, during which the exercises are repeated—this type of work, combined with weakness in the stabilizer muscles around the ankle, often creates acute trauma in the ankle. These can range from light injuries to a full tear of the ankle ligaments and will mostly occur in inversion movements.

Due to an ankle sprain being widely considered a mild injury, there exists a tendency not to treat it professionally with the help of an expert. This is one reason we often observe recurring sprains and ankle muscle weakness in gymnasts.

11.6.4 Prevention

The literature supports prevention as the best treatment in high-level CAI (chronic ankle instability) athletes.

Several high-quality studies have demonstrated the beneficial effects of proprioceptive training on unstable surfaces in reducing the risk of ankle sprains, improving ankle stability and preventing re-sprains such as the prospective controlled trial by Verhagen et al. [6] and the cohort study by Doherty et al. [7]. Recently, it was also shown that rhythmic gymnasts improved their dynamic postural balance after a period of 8 weeks of proprioceptive exercise training.

Also, several studies suggest that the retinacula of the ankle, which is an aponeurotic fascia, innervated by a large number of mechanoreceptors and free nerve endings, thus plays an important role in proprioception of the ankle, preventing ankle sprains and injuries. Fascial manipulation® can improve ankle proprioception, range of motion, and stability, which may reduce the risk of sprains and other ankle injuries. Other studies, such as the randomized controlled trial by Brandolini et al. [8], have found that interventions that target the fascia and retinacula, such as Fascial Manipulation® therapy, can be effective in preventing chronic ankle instability and improving overall ankle function. These findings suggest that treating the retinacula and fascia may be an important component of ankle injury prevention and rehabilitation protocols.

This is why we, at the Israeli Rhythmic Gymnastics National Team, have incorporated three components of prevention into the daily training program, as part of a sprain-prevention program. One is strengthening of the foot muscles using TheraBand as part of foot warmup.

Balance and neuro-muscular control represents an important part of gymnasts warmup and are performed on a balance platform or balance disc, and includes one-leg stands, without looking, all during functional handheld apparatus work. Additionally, some of the practice on balance and fitness elements is also performed on unstable surfaces. Gymnasts who need additional practice also perform similar exercises (on unstable surfaces, strengthening foot, knee, and thigh stabilizers) at the end of the session.

As part of the weekly physiotherapy sessions that gymnasts undergo, they receive (at least once per month) a fascial manipulation treatment around the ankle, specifically the retinacula, in order to prevent injuries.

11.6.5 Notes for Rehabilitation

The same methods for prevention we use also in the rehabilitation process.

It is important to highlight the importance of utilizing functional exercises in the rehabilitation of elite gymnasts, thus providing them exercises without relying on the visual system with a hand apparatus during specific rhythmic gymnastics elements.

11.6.6 Achilles Tendinopathy

The incidence of Achilles tendinopathy is high in young female gymnasts (17.5%). It was hypothesized that specific elements in that sports activity are responsible for muscle overload of gastrocnemius-soleus group [9].

Risk factors for the development of Achilles tendinopathy in rhythmic gymnasts include the frequency and intensity of training—during most of the training, the gymnast stands on her toes (*relevé*) together with the combination of significant shortening in the gastrocnemius-soleus muscles and insufficient stretching and releasing those muscle groups between training sessions [10].

During periods when a gymnast has a growth spurt and is significantly taller, it seems that in addition to pain that could appear in the insertion of the patellar tendon, it is also very typical to see pain in the insertion of the Achilles tendon—usually it will appear bilaterally.

11.6.7 Prevention

Incorporation of stretching exercises of the gastrocnemius and soleus muscle group into every practice (passive and dynamic stretching of the muscles behind the shin area, with both a straight and bent knee), during warmup and also after the session. At the start of every session, as part of the warmup, release the muscles behind the entire shin and thigh area by using a foam roller and then rolling a small ball over the plantar arch. The attention should be guided toward releasing the entire back of the leg and not just to the back of the shin and Achilles area.

11.6.8 Notes for Rehabilitation

From many years of experience working with gymnasts, I noticed that at the acute stage of the pain, much faster results are obtained when the gymnast focuses on *self-release* (using a roller) *or by manual treatment done by a professional* at the back area of the shin, the plantar fascia, and the hamstring area. Only several days later, when the pain starts to fade away, can she start to *stretch* the gastrocnemius. This is done to relieve the pressure without further stimulating the insertion area of the Achilles tendon. Obviously, it is recommended to begin with physiotherapy and manual treatments as soon as possible to relieve local pain and release tissues.

11.6.9 Knee Injuries

Several studies have reported a 19.1% of prevalence of knee pain and knee problems in rhythmic gymnasts [11]. The main pain is patellofemoral pain, followed by the medial and lateral menisci. The incidence of patellofemoral pain and functional outcome in rhythmic gymnasts is similar to the general population; the sport practice does not trigger patellofemoral pain [11]. Moreover, limb and hindfoot alignment seems to be not particularly involved in the symptomatology. Low incidence of patellofemoral pain in gymnasts could be related to the training modality, characterized by a high-flexibility training program, compared to other high-impact sports [12]. As described earlier in the chapter about the special characteristics of the sport, knee hyperextension is a key factor that receives great attention in the field. Gymnasts are required to reach hyperextension in the knees in every element they perform, some of which include leaning and standing on one leg for extensive time periods. These elements are where gymnasts often complain about patellofemoral pains.

Another common phenomenon appearing in many gymnasts is a medial collapse of the knee (knee valgus or valgus collapse) during landing or leaning over the knees. This is commonly accompanied by a medial collapse of the foot (pes planus). In such cases, gymnasts will largely point to pains in the medial section of the knee and describe pains mostly while landing from jumps.

11.6.10 Prevention

To prevent knee injuries in this population, proper training techniques and injury prevention strategies should be implemented. To avoid frontal knee pains in one-leg stands, it is important to train the gymnasts to use the quad muscles, the hip stabilizers, and the core, and to not passively decline into knee hyperextensions (which most gymnasts do due to hypermobility).

For most scenarios, teaching the correct technique prevents pain. To relieve medial knee pains in landings, the key is to start from the foot. Most gymnasts have a pes planus in the foot arch (reasons for that are described in the previous chapter). This leads to a medial collapse of the knee (valgus collapse) and creates inadequate mechanical load on the medial section of the knee—followed by pains. The way to prevent this is to train the gymnast to actively lift the foot arch and use the external rotators of the thigh and knee, in order to place the knee over the second or third toe line in landings and in any contraction of the knee—thus avoiding medial collapse. After training, it is beneficial to assign a functional exercise (landings, balance, one-leg elements) using a resistance band (the band pulls the knee into internal rotation) in which the gymnast must keep the knee in the proper position. It is also recommended to add strengthening exercises for the thigh and hip stabilizers.

Another key point in preventing knee injuries is using protective equipment the use of knee pads in practice will protect the knees and can relieve knee pains caused by prolonged leaning on the knees.

11.6.11 Notes for Rehabilitation

In addition to physiotherapy and manual treatment, it is worth paying attention to assigning functional exercises, as close as possible to the usual exercises that the gymnast performs. As mentioned earlier, every gymnast performs unique elements, and the rehabilitation and the building of correct technique should be based on those same elements in order to allow her to implement the corrections best (Fig. 11.5).

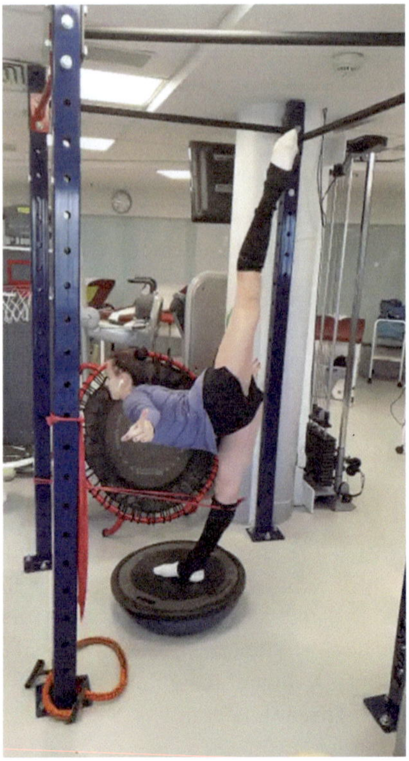

Fig. 11.5 Functional exercise for knee rehabilitation on an unstable surface." © Photograph by "Natalie Brettler". All rights reserved. Reproduced with permissions

11.6.12 Thigh Injuries

Several studies have reported a high prevalence of hip pain and injuries in rhythmic gymnasts due to the repetitive and specific nature of their training that involves combinations of extreme hip flexion, extension, abduction, and external rotation, muscular imbalances, and side-to-side differences. The hip/groin is the third most frequently reported location of injury and pain after the feet and the back. Common hip injuries reported include labral tears, femur-acetabular impingement (FAI), hip flexor strains, and hip adductor strains, These injuries can have a significant impact on the gymnast's performance and the elements they can perform [14]. Rhythmic gymnasts are very similar to professional ballet dancers in their hip injuries as their movements are very similar.

11.6.13 Dysplasia and Instability

Increased hip ROM that is required in rhythmic gymnastics can be also the outcome of hyperlaxity and/or hip dysplasia. Research has shown that dancers with both hyperlaxity and dysplasia have sustained low-energy hip dislocations during dance [19]. Hammond et al. [21] found that 55% of professional dancers undergoing hip arthroscopy for labral pathology had evidence of dysplasia.

11.7 Labral Tears and Impingement

Femur-acetabular impingement (FAI) syndrome is a motion-related clinical disorder of the hip with a triad of symptoms, clinical signs, and imaging findings. It represents symptomatic premature contact between the proximal femur and the acetabulum. The pain is reported in the groin or hip but also in the lateral hip, anterior thigh, buttock, knee, lower back, and lateral and posterior thigh [20]. Symptomatic (FAI) could be due to pathoanatomy of pincer-type FAI (more common in dancers) or cam-type FAI [15], but it can be also secondary to the repetitive training and compensatory soft tissue laxity driven from extreme ROM of hyperextension/hyperflexion and external rotation/abduction. FAI could also create impingement-induced subluxation at the posterior-superior aspect of the hip, corresponding with the cartilage thinning and labral pathology often seen on hip MRI of asymptomatic dancers and in cadaveric studies [16]. Those studies also show that combinations of hip abduction and external rotation in both flexion and extension cause increased labral strain and anterior femoral head subluxation (Fig. 11.6).

Several types of extra-articular impingement could occur: trochanteric-pelvic impingement or an extra-articular bony impingement between the anterior inferior iliac spine (AIIS) and distal femoral neck (subspinous impingement) in extreme hip flexion, either neutral rotation or abduction [17]. Another type is ischiofemoral impingement—between the lesser trochanter and the ischium in positions of hip extension, adduction, and external rotation. The symptoms will be in

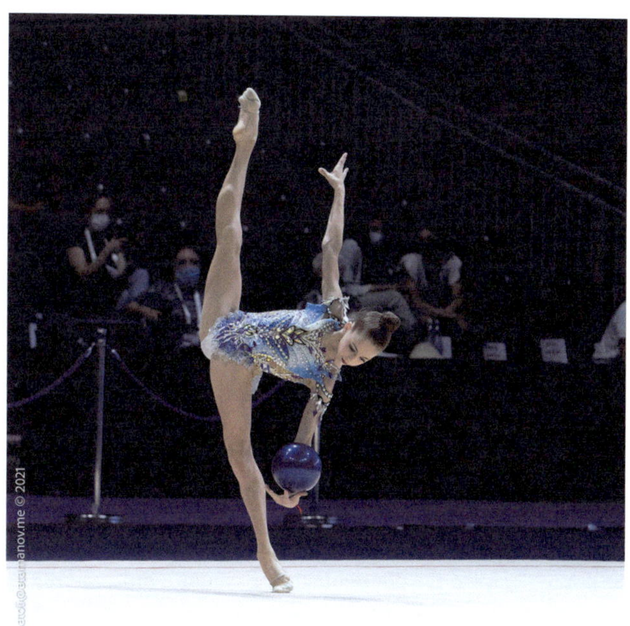

Fig. 11.6 Femoroacetabular impingement (FAI) can be secondary to repetitive training involving extreme ranges of motion, including hyperextension, hyperflexion, and external rotation/abduction of the hip- basic elements in rhythmic gymnastics." © Photograph by "Anatoli Atamanov". All rights reserved. Reproduced with permissions

the groin and/or buttocks and may be felt similar to hamstring strain [18].

A rhythmic gymnast can have also a combination of instability and impingement; usually the retroverted dysplastic acetabulum will cause anterior impingement but posterior-superior instability.

11.7.1 Prevention

It is recommended that rhythmic gymnasts receive regular hip screening by a physical therapist and appropriate preventative measures, such as targeted strengthening exercises, to reduce the risk of hip injuries.

As a preventative program, The Takla-O'Donnell Protocol (TOP) could be used for strengthening of the deep hip muscles to facilitate local muscular control followed by global retraining.

Moreover, many gymnasts complain of pain during the Penche' rotation. Some of them do not perform this element with the correct technique—instead of using the abdominal, back, and pelvic muscles in order to stabilize their body in this element, they collapse into the excessive flexibility of the hip and rely on the flexibility of the hip joint. Many times, by learning the correct technique and practicing it, the hip pain in these elements decreases.

11.7.2 Notes for Rehabilitation

Physiotherapist-led rehabilitation should aim to reduce the gymnast's symptoms by improving first of all hip stability (recommended by the Takla-O'Donnell Protocol), neuromuscular control, and movement patterns and to correct technique if needed. If the conservative treatment didn't work, an operation can be a solution. For the most part, these gymnasts will not undergo surgery because of the long rehabilitation involved and will choose conservative treatment or not to perform the elements that create the hip symptoms.

11.7.3 Muscle Strain

As mentioned above, one of the most important criteria on which the gymnast is judged is the flexibility of the hips. The extreme ROM requirements and the repetitive pattern in this sport could cause muscle strain around the hip, usually in hip flexors, adductors, and extensors. Previous research also suggested that muscle strains are more prevalent in older adolescent gymnasts, whereas strains in early adolescence occur near ossification centers. It's important to note that muscle strains could also occur from the passive stretching that the coaches tend to do to gymnasts to increase their flexibility.

11.8 Prevention

Consistent physiotherapy and specifically manual treatment or self-release using a roller, not only when in pain but also regularly, can prevent or decrease the frequency and severity of such muscle injuries. Another point for prevention is a gradual warmup, static and dynamic, at the start of every practice session. Due to many gymnasts being endowed with hypermobility, most of them arrive at practice and sit down in a split right away, with no gradual warmup of the joint. At a young age, this normally will not lead to any injury, but at older ages, a non-gradual, steep warmup increases the risk of muscle and joint injuries. Many gymnasts report that using a roller to dynamically release the muscle at the start of the warmup allows them to stretch and warm up with ease.

11.9 Notes for Rehabilitation

The rehabilitation should include physical therapy and myofascial treatments [21]. Beyond those, it is important to emphasize the importance of muscular rehabilitation in creating strength at the end of the ranges as required by the gymnast in the gymnastics elements.

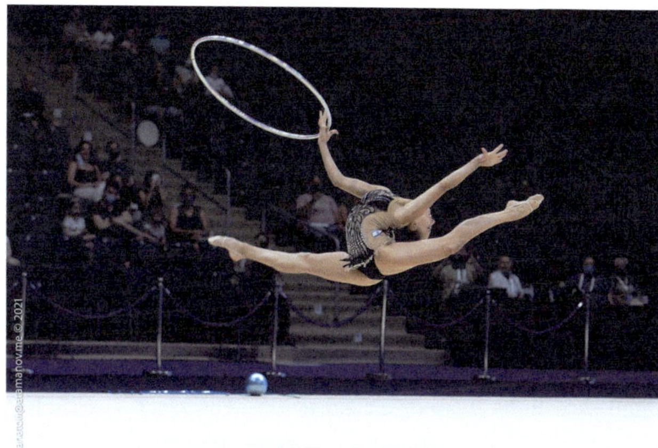

Fig. 11.7 Rhythmic gymnast performing a leap with a deep spinal arch while manipulating the hoop apparatus. Repeated extreme lumbar hyperextension, as seen in this movement, may contribute to the development of low back injuries in rhythmic gymnasts." © Photograph by "Anatoli Atamanov". All rights reserved. Reproduced with permissions

11.9.1 Back Injuries

Rhythmic gymnastics provides a high-risk environment for developing lower-back pain and injuries due to the intense physical demands of the sport, which include repeated extreme hyperflexion and hyperextension and asymmetric repetitive elements that are required for RG. The incidence rate of spinal problems in rhythmic gymnastics varies in articles between 19% and 80% [22]. These injuries can range from minor muscle strains to more severe conditions such as spondylolysis and spondylolisthesis (Fig 11.7).

11.10 Muscle Strains, Spondylolysis, and Spondylolisthesis

There is a high incidence of spondylolysis among gymnasts with low-back pain. Spondylolysis and spondylolisthesis are more common in rhythmic gymnasts than the normal population, with spondylolysis affecting approximately 8% of the normal population but up to 20% of rhythmic gymnasts. Therefore, the medical staff have to be very suspicious when a gymnast develops such symptoms, especially when the pain is located exactly in the middle of the spine and not relieved by treatments and occurs on every extension of the back and landing from jumps. Many authors have attributed the high rate of spondylolysis among gymnasts and dancers to increased lordosis and dynamic hyperextension of the spine.

Lumbar disc bulges are rare, and it is more common to see facet joint dysfunctions.

Spondylolisthesis is a translation of one vertebra on another. Gymnasts are more likely to have an isthmic spondylolisthesis—an anterolisthesis resulting from bilateral spondylolysis lesions. Low-grade symptomatic spondylolisthesis may be managed conservatively, and management strategies may be similar to that for spondylolysis [27].

11.10.1 Prevention

Proper conditioning, strengthening exercises, and injury prevention strategies can help reduce the incidence of back injuries in rhythmic gymnasts. Early detection and proper management of any back pain and injury can help prevent further damage and allow athletes to continue competing at a high level [23, 25].

Prevention of back pain consists of three main components:

Warmup, with gradual dynamic stretching and gradual increase in techniques.

Strengthening of the abdominal, back, and pelvic stabilizers.

Balancing the training as possible between the right and left sides of the body.

Releasing muscles and fascia as a treatment but also prophylactically.

From my clinical experience, gymnasts may suffer from back pain and indeed need a specific release of the back, but many times, releasing other areas will cause the pain to decrease. The Olympic champion (Tokyo 2020) Linoy Ashram, who was treated by me in the years of her senior career, suffered from lower-back pain in the last year before the Olympic Games. In the MRI, a small disc bulge was observed at L5. The treatment that helped her the most was a myofascial release in the neck and feet. Touching her directly on her lower back made her pain worse. A bilateral myofascial release of the adductor muscles of the hip will reduce back pain for some, while there are those who get a relief from a myofascial release of the front chains (iliopsoas, quads and tibialis anterior) in the lower back. The treatment should be adapted to the gymnast according to the elements she performs in the exercises and the characteristics of her body.

11.11 Notes for Rehabilitation

The most important is early recognition of a developing spondylolytic lesion. When diagnosed by clinical symptoms and the appearance of the lesion on CT, the gymnast should stop immediately back extension movements, jumps, and any other movement that manifest pain in the back for a 12-week period or until the symptoms resolve. During this period, the gymnasts enter a phase of rehabilitation. They are allowed to participate in trainings and work on strengthening and stabilization exercises and apparatus handling. Aerobic fitness can be saved by swimming on the back. All of them should be pain-free without load on the spine. Rehabilitation of spondylolysis as well as other overuse syndromes of the posterior elements of the spine should involve specific exercises to increase abdominal strength and improve hamstring and lumbodorsal fascia flexibility and anti-lordotic postural exercise.

Successful return to full practice can be expected only after the gymnast has achieved all goals of the rehabilitation program, can accomplish full and pain-free range of motion, has adequate strength and aerobic fitness, and is able to perform sport-specific skills without pain.

11.11.1 Scoliosis

Scoliosis often develops just prior to and during puberty. There is a tenfold-higher incidence of scoliosis in gymnasts compared with controls, which has been suggested to be due to their increased ligament laxity, dysmenorrhea, and asymmetrical loading of gymnastics training.

11.12 Prevention

Probably the only thing we can influence in the context of scoliosis in gymnasts is the symmetrical practice. Many gymnasts place considerable emphasis on developing and strengthening the dominant leg and thus do not adhere to symmetrical practice in training. While during their exercise the practice cannot be symmetrical, they should make sure to practice symmetrically in the warmup, ballet, and during strengthening exercises.

11.13 Notes for Rehabilitation

Schroth scoliosis-specific exercises have demonstrated promising results in reducing the progression of scoliosis and reducing the Cobb angle [24] and, therefore, may be considered for use also with rhythmic gymnasts.

11.13.1 Shoulder Injuries

The percentage of injuries of the upper limbs in rhythmic gymnastics is very low, described in the various studies between 1% and 6% and will be mainly either overuse, muscle strains, or shoulder dislocation [22]. A rhythmic gymnast hardly carries any weight on her hands (apart from simple acrobatic elements such as a cartwheel or handstand (but performs a lot of elements that demand strength and flexibility of the shoulder joint (difficult grips outside the visual range). That is why the injuries that occur are more muscle overuse injuries since the gymnast must work non-stop with the hand apparatus or shoulder dislocation due to the hyper flexibility elements that are required with the apparatus. Every gymnast has a dominant hand, but working with the apparatus must be done almost equally in both hands in the exercise.

11.13.2 Prevention

The main prevention relies in physical therapy and maintaining regular myofascial release together with exercises for the stabilizers of the shoulders and the wrist.

11.14 Notes for Rehabilitation

In case of shoulder dislocation, usually the treatment will be conservative physical therapy rehabilitation, as most of the gymnasts are with hyperlaxity and success in surgery in this situation is generally less predictable [26].

References

1. Zhu M, Arai N, Ueji M, Hayakawa I, Inokuchi S, Tagami K. Cross-sectional view of foot growth and deformity in young Japanese rhythmic gymnasts. Bull Facul Health Sci. 2015;38:23–31.
2. Kim MH, Kwon OY, Kim SH, et al. Comparison of muscle activities of abductor hallucis and adductor hallucis between the short foot and toespread- out exercises in subjects with mild hallux valgus. J Back Musculoskeletal Rehabil. 2013;26:163–8.
3. Kim MK, Jeon HS, Kim TH. Effect of toe-spread-out exercise on hallux valgus angle and cross-sectional area of abductor hallucis muscle in subjects with hallux valgus. J Phys Ther Sci. 2015;27(4):1019–22.
4. Sarwark JF. Essentials of musculoskeletal care. 4th ed. Illinois: American Academy of Orthopaedic Surgeons; 2010.
5. Oltean A, Rusu MM, Copoiu N, Calin MF. Incidence of injuries in rhythmic gymnastics. Sci Movement Health. 2017a;17(2, Supplement):427–32.
6. Verhagen E, van der Beek A, Twisk J, Bouter L, Bahr R, van Mechelen W. The effect of a proprioceptive balance board training program for the prevention of ankle sprains: a prospective controlled trial. Am J Sports Med. 2004;32(6):1385–93. https://doi.org/10.1177/0363546503262177.
7. Doherty C, Delahunt E, Caulfield B, Hertel J, Ryan J, Bleakley C, Hiller C. The incidence and prevalence of ankle sprain injury: a systematic review and meta-analysis of prospective epidemiological studies. Sports Med. 2014;44(1):123–40. https://doi.org/10.1007/s40279-013-0102-5.
8. Brandolini S, Lugaresi G, Santagata A, Ermolao A, Zaccaria M, Marchand A, Stecco A. Sport injury prevention in individuals with chronic ankle instability: fascial manipulation® versus control group: a randomized controlled trial. J Bodyw Mov Ther. 2019;23(4):742–9.
9. Notarnicola A, Maccagnano G, Di Leo M, Tafuri S, Moretti B. Overload and neovascularization of Achilles tendons in young artistic and rhythmic gymnasts compared with controls: an observational study. Musculoskelet Surg. 2014;98(2):115–20.
10. Thevendran G, Sarraf KM, Patel NK, Sadri A, Rosenfeld P. The ruptured Achilles tendon: a current overview from biology of rupture to treatment. Musculoskelet Surg. 2013;97(1):9–20.
11. Cupisti A, D'Alessandro C, Evangelisti I, Unbri C, Rossi M, Galetta F, Panicucci E, Lopes Pegna S, Piazza M. Injury survey in competitive subelite rhythmic gymnasts: results from a prospective controlled study. J Sports Med Phys Fitness. 2007;47:203–7.
12. Pavone V, Vescio A, Panvini FMC, Lucenti L, Testa G, Sessa G. Patellofemoral pain syndrome in young female athletes: a case-control study. Adv Orthoped. 2022;17:2022.
13. Oltean A, Rusu MM, Copoiu N, Călin MF. Incidence of injuries in rhythmic gymnastics. Ovidius Univer Ann Phys Educ Sport Sci. 2017b;17(2):427–32.
14. Bolia I, Utsunomiya H, Locks R, Briggs K, Philippon MJ. Twenty-year systematic review of the hip pathology, risk factors, treatment, and clinical outcomes in artistic athletes – dancers, figure skaters, and gymnasts. Clin J Sport Med. 2018;28:82–90.
15. Sink EL, Gralla J, Ryba A, Dayton M. Clinical presentation of femoroacetabular impingement in adolescents. J Pediatr Orthop. 2008;28:806–11.
16. Dy CJ, Thompson MT, Crawford MJ, Alexander JW, McCarthy JC, Noble PC. Tensile strain in the anterior part of the acetabular labrum during provocative maneuvering of the normal hip. J Bone Joint Surg Am. 2008;90:1464–72.
17. Larson CM, Kelly BT, Stone RM. Making a case for anterior inferior iliac spine/subspine hip impingement: three representative case reports and proposed concept. Arthroscopy. 2011;27:1732–7.
18. Besomi J, Garin A, Herrera C, Maffiuletti NA. Ischiofemoral impingement in adolescents: from

clinical presentation to return to sports. Orthop J Sports Med. 2019;7(1)
19. Epstein DM, Rose DJ, Philippon MJ. Arthroscopic management of recurrent low-energy anterior hip dislocation in a dancer: a case report and review of literature. Am J Sports Med. 2010;38:1250–4.
20. Griffin DR, Dickenson EJ, O'Donnell J, Agricola R, Awan T, Beck M, et al. The Warwick agreement on femoroacetabular impingement syndrome (FAI syndrome): an international consensus statement. Br J Sports Med. 2016;50(19):1169–76.
21. Hammond KE, Kneer L, Vopat BG. Rehabilitation of soft tissue injuries of the hip and pelvis. Clin Sports Med. 2021;40(1):115–29. https://doi.org/10.1016/j.csm.2020.08.011.
22. Caine D, Knutzen K, Howe W, Keeler L, Sheppard L, Henrichs D, Fast J. A three-year epidemiological study of injuries affecting young female gymnasts. Phys Ther Sport. 2003;4(1):10–23.
23. Miguel A, Simões V, Pizzari T, Ford JJ. A profile of the characteristics of back pain in young adult rhythmic gymnasts: a prospective observational study. Phys Ther Sport. 2019;40:66–71. https://doi.org/10.1016/j.ptsp.2019.06.007.
24. Burger M, Coetzee W, du Plessis LZ, Geldenhuys L, Joubert F, Myburgh E, van Rooyen C, Vermeulen N. The effectiveness of Schroth exercises in adolescents with idiopathic scoliosis: a systematic review and meta-analysis. S Afr J Physiother. 2019;75(1):904.
25. Micheli LJ, Solomon R. Back pain in young athletes. Am J Lifestyle Med. 2019;13(4):386–91. https://doi.org/10.1177/1559827618769812.
26. Rupp MC, Rutledge JC, Quinn PM, Millett PJ. Management of shoulder instability in patients with underlying hyperlaxity. Curr Rev Musculoskelet Med. 2023;16:1–10.
27. Cavalier R, Herman MJ, Cheung EV, et al. Spondylolysis and spondylolisthesis in children and adolescents: I. Diagnosis, natural history, and nonsurgical management. J Am Acad Orthop Surg. 2006;14:417Y24.

Snowboarding

12

Francesco Feletti, Nicola Pegoraro, and Aldo Carnevale

12.1 Introduction

Snowboarding is a popular winter recreational and competitive activity where participants descend snow-covered slopes while standing on a board fixed to their feet. It emerged in the 1960s and 1970s in the United States, drawing inspiration from skateboarding, sledging, surfing, and skiing [1].

The first snowboard was constructed in 1965 by Sherman Poppen, an engineer in Muskegon, Michigan, who invented a prototype called the "snurfer". It consisted of two snow skis attached, with a rope at the front for steering.

This innovative design laid the foundation for the modern snowboard, and soon, a sports equipment manufacturer, Brunswick Corporation, licensed it and began producing and distributing it nationwide.

Local Michigan snuffers competition followed in the late 1960s, spreading to national competitions in the 1970s.

In 1975, surfer Dimitrije Milovich evolved the initial snowboard design into a similar modern longboard [2]. This evolution sparked the advent of new inventors and pioneers like Burton, Sims, and Barfoot, who introduced innovative technologies and established manufacturing companies. They also played a crucial role in organizing the first official snowboard competitions, such as the National Snow Surfing Championships in 1982 and the World Championship Halfpipe Competition in 1983 [3].

After a few years of general difficult acceptance, snowboarding grew in popularity: at first, the competitions were races like skiing but soon evolved into freestyle events.

Finally, in 1994, the International Olympic Committee (IOC) officially recognized snowboarding as a sport, debuting it at the 1998 Winter Games in Nagano, Japan, with men's and women's giant slalom and halfpipe competitions. Since then, various disciplines have been added to the Olympic program, including snowboard cross, slopestyle, and big air [3].

In 2014, the International Paralympic Committee introduced adaptive snowboarding

F. Feletti (✉)
Dipartimento di Medicina Traslazionale e per la Romagna, Università di Ferrara, Ferrara, Italy

Unità Operativa di Radiologia, Ospedale S. Maria delle Croci, Ausl della Romagna, Ravenna, Italy

EXTREMESPORTMED, International Society of Medicine for Outdoor Physical Activity and Extreme Sports, Città Metropolitana di Bologna, Bologna, Italy
e-mail: francesco.feletti@unife.it

N. Pegoraro · A. Carnevale
Dipartimento di Medicina Traslazionale e per la Romagna, Università di Ferrara, Ferrara, Italy

Unità Operativa di Radiologia, Arcispedale S. Anna, Aosp Ferrara, Cona, Ferrara, Italy
e-mail: nicola01.pegoraro@edu.unife.it; aldo.carnevale@unife.it

H. Jones, A. Lukaszenko (eds.), *Injury Prevention and Care in Artistic Sports*,
https://doi.org/10.1007/978-3-032-18105-3_12

("para-snowboarding") at the Paralympic Winter Games in Sochi.

Snowboarding has evolved into distinct and unique styles, each with its equipment, terrain, and methods, with a variable overlap. Freestyle, freeride, and free carve/race are now popular subgenres.

12.1.1 Freestyle

Freestyle snowboarding identifies the most creative qualities of the sport. It is defined as using natural and artificial elements such as rails, jumps, and other obstacles to perform aerial movements and tricks. Competitive freestyle riding can be classified into halfpipe/superpipe, slopestyle, Big Air, and rail jams [4].

Freestyle riders typically choose a shorter snowboard to provide the flexibility and mobility required to complete their skills (Fig. 12.1).

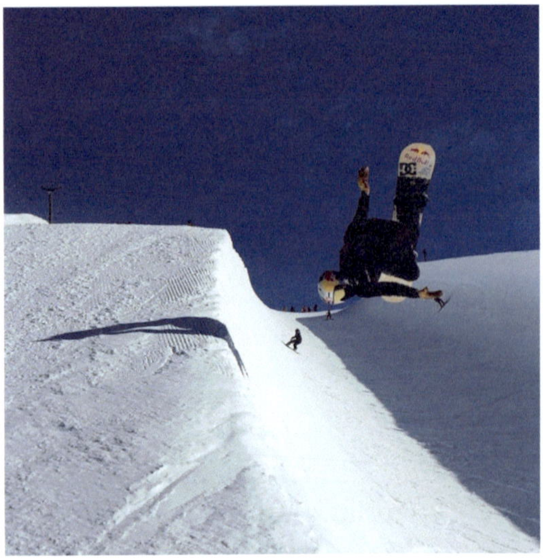

Fig. 12.1 Big Air. (Photo by Markos Mant; Innsbruck, Austria)

The halfpipe, snowboarding's most famous competition, is held in a half-tube of snow with slopes of around 18°, where athletes perform tricks while moving from one side to the other and launching into the air above the edges (Fig. 12.2).

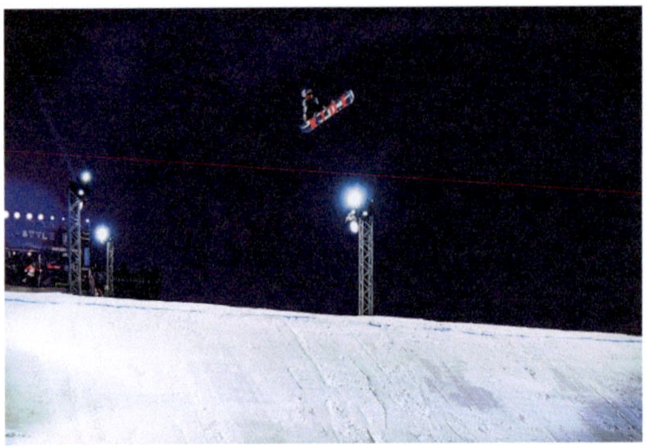

Fig. 12.2 Halfpipe. (Photo by Rowan Simpson; Cardrona Alpine Resort Cardrona Valley Rd., Cardrona, New Zealand)

Superpipe has higher walls and approximately 90-degree vertical walls, although an official definition does not exist.

In slopestyle, athletes execute tricks by going around, over, and across various terrain obstacles and jumping throughout a course.

Big Air events are contests where riders perform tricks in the air after launching off a jump before a clean landing (Fig. 12.3).

Rail jams are held in diverse locations, incorporating rail-type features and urban-style elements, allowing competitors to showcase their creativity (Fig. 12.4).

12.1.2 Freeriding

Freeriding emphasizes utilizing natural terrain and challenging nature's obstacles without constructed impediments. It is often practiced in the backcountry and big mountain settings, where riders seek extreme and untouched locations.

12.1.3 Free Carve/Race

Alpine snowboarding, or free carving, is often practiced on groomed courses and focuses on carving linked turns. It shares similarities with skiing, particularly in its slalom variants, where the priority is slicing around offset poles, or "gates", at high speeds.

Snowboard cross is a snowboarding variant in which many riders compete head to head down a

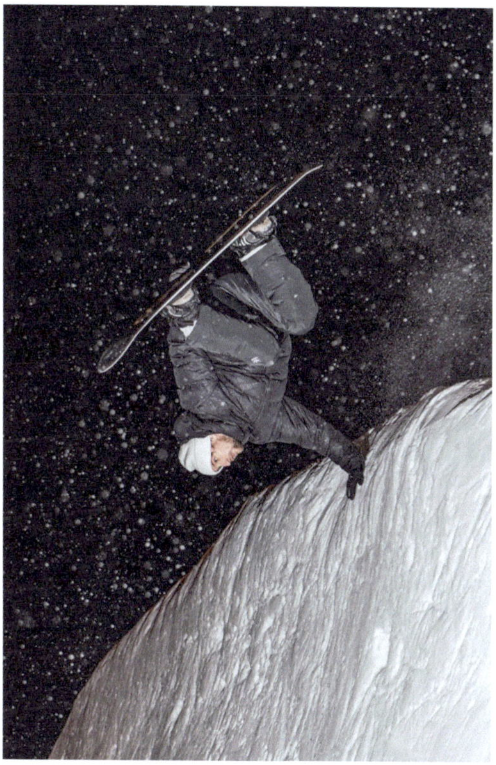

Fig. 12.3 Freestyle trick. (Photo by Ilya Shishikhin; Ruka, Финляндия)

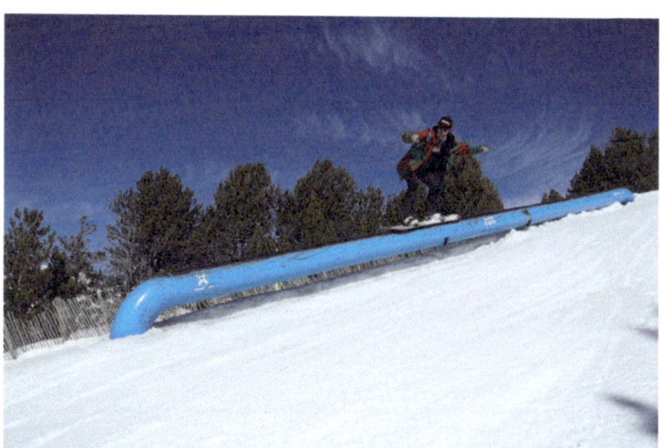

Fig. 12.4 Rail Jam. (Photo by Andrii Denysenko)

course that includes jumps, berms, and other obstacles to test balance and control at high speed to finish the race first.

Various national and international associations have played a vital role in developing and establishing the sport. The International Snowboarding Federation, an organization formed to oversee snowboarding competitions, helped promote snowboarding as an Olympic sport in the 1998 Winter Olympics [5]. However, the International Olympic Committee recognized the International Ski Federation (FIS) as the legitimate governing organization of the sport.

In 2022, FIS changed its name to "International Ski and Snowboard Federation", confirming its position as the leading international regulatory body for skiing and snowboarding, including Olympic competition standards.

The United States of America Snowboarding and Freeski Association (USASA) also plays an influential role, offering grassroots tournaments that serve as stepping stones for young athletes looking to advance in the competitive pipeline.

Beyond the Olympic Games, there are other well-renowned events, like the X Games, an annual competition that expresses the real extreme nature of the sport, the Freeride World Tour, the FIS World Cup, and the FIS World Championships, which include Big Air, halfpipe, slalom subtypes, slopestyle, and snowboard cross for both genders, as well as mixed team events [6].

There have been many influential and famous snowboarders throughout the sport's history.

Shaun White is perhaps the most famous snowboarder of all time. He gained widespread recognition for his incredible talent and dominance in halfpipe and slopestyle competitions. White won multiple Olympic gold medals and X Games titles, solidifying his status as a snowboarding legend [7].

Chloe Kim burst onto the snowboarding scene with her impressive skills and infectious personality. At 17, she became the youngest woman to win an Olympic snowboarding gold medal in the halfpipe at the 2018 Winter Olympics [8].

Terje Haakonsen is widely regarded as one of the most influential snowboarders in history. Known for his progressive riding style, he was a dominant force in the 1990s, winning numerous halfpipe and big air competitions [9].

These snowboarders attained fame through their exceptional skills and competitive achievements and are among those who have most contributed to the progression of snowboarding as an international and Olympic sport.

12.2 Specificities of the Sport/Art

Freestyle snowboarding is the discipline that genuinely expresses the aesthetic and artistic aspect of the sport, where the focus lies on delivering a captivating show and executing spectacular and challenging tricks.

Competitions are typically practiced on purpose-built slopes and halfpipes, precisely designed for an event. However, in the backcountry freestyle version, tricks are performed in remote locations, on off-piste routes, and include extreme jumps from ridges and rocks, adding an even more breath-taking element to the sport.

There are various types of tricks on snowboarding that are all rooted in ollies and nollies.

The ollie technique aims to lift the board off the ground by propelling oneself into the air and balancing the weight backwards. Typically, this is achieved by utilizing obstacles or ramps and jumping off their edges [10].

The nollie technique is used in specific rail tricks and follows a similar principle but with a slight variation: the pop is directed forward instead of straight up by shifting the weight forward and then using the board's nose (or toe) to take flight [11].

The snowboarding tricks can be categorized into four main groups: Butter, Grab, Spin and Flip [10].

Butter tricks revolve around board movement and control. They include tricks such as the 180 nose roll and 180 tail drag. These tricks involve initiating a turn with either the nose or tail of the board, lifting the board while keeping the respective end (nose or tail) in contact with the snow, and then spinning the board to land in a switch (reverse) stance. The 360 versions of these tricks require more momentum and rotational force, with a complete 360-degree rotation performed in the air.

Grab tricks occur when the rider holds the board with their hand during a jump. There are various types of grabs, each named after the part of the board that is grabbed and the hand used. For example, an Indy grab involves reaching down and grabbing the heel edge of the board between the bindings with the rear hand. Other popular grabs include the Nose grab, Tail grab, Mute grab, and Stalefish grab [12]. Grab tricks add style and creativity to jumps, and the longer the grab is held, the more impressive the manoeuvre becomes.

Spin tricks involve rotations along the horizontal axis while in the air during a jump. These tricks can range from 180 half spins to 360 full spins and even more complex multiple rotations like the 540, 720, 900, and 1080. Depending on the rider's stance, spins can be executed in a frontside or backside direction. Adding a grab to a spin increases the difficulty level and enhances the visual appeal of the trick [12].

Flip tricks encompass vertical rotations that can be performed forward or backward [11]. The most well-known flip trick is the backflip, which involves rotating backwards in the air and landing. Front flips, which are forward rotations, are popular but require high skill and control. Flips can be combined with grabs, adding extra difficulty and style. However, due to the increased risk of landing on the head or neck, flips are considered highly dangerous and should only be attempted by experienced and trained riders [11].

These tricks, including grabs, spins, and flips, are just a glimpse into the world of freestyle snowboarding. They represent the creativity, athleticism, and technical skill required to push the boundaries of the sport. Riders continue to innovate and create new tricks, adding to the ever-evolving and thrilling nature of freestyle snowboarding.

12.3 Epidemiology of More Frequent Injuries

The knowledge of sport-specific injury dynamics in extreme sports is critical for the development of effective preparation, rehabilitation, and safety systems [13].

Among recreational snowboarders, an overall injury rate (IR) of 4–16 injuries per 1000 snowboarder days was reported [14].

Major et al. [15] calculated the injury rate (IR) in the cohort of elite FIS World Cup (WC) snowboarders by defining injuries as "all acute injuries that occurred during training or competition and required attention by medical personnel".

The overall IR was 40.1 injuries per 100 athletes per season. During the FIS WC competitions, an IR of 6.4 injuries/1000 runs was calculated; it was highest in snowboard cross, reaching values of 11.9/1000 runs, followed by 6.3 in halfpipe, 3.6 in big air, and 2.8 in parallel giant slalom/parallel slalom.

Snowboard cross also presented the highest risk of severe injuries (>28 days absence).

A significant number of snow sports enthusiasts now frequent snow parks, even if only occasionally. Epidemiological studies suggest that the likelihood of accidents in these facilities is higher than on traditional slopes, much like in commercial skateparks, where, despite mandatory safety equipment, injuries tend to be more frequent due to heightened competition and a preference for riskier riding styles [16, 17].

In snowboarding, the most common types of injuries are fractures (31.7%), strains and sprains (25.2%), contusions (10.9%), and concussions (10.0%) [18].

In particular, recreational snowboarders are widely accepted to be at an increased risk of head and upper arm injuries.

Among snowboarding participants, wrist sprains or fractures are the most commonly reported injuries, representing around 44% of all upper-extremity injuries and 21.6% of all snowboarding injuries [19].

Additionally, forearm and shoulder joint injuries are common, accounting for 22.5% and 19.3% of the upper extremity injuries, respectively [18].

Ankle and foot injuries, including sprains and fractures, are common in snowboarders, representing 17.1% of all injuries [20].

Snowboarders encounter a high risk of spinal and head injuries, particularly among beginners and in halfpipe and big air variants [21, 22].

The lumbar spine represents the most commonly injured site, with 34.5–69.4% of spinal injuries [22].

Traumatic brain concussions are the most common winter sports injury requiring hospital admission, and often subdural hematoma is the main complication that occurs [23].

Also, abdominal injuries can occur, caused by blunt force to the posterolateral and flank regions, primarily affecting the retroperitoneal organs, with the risk of splenic and kidney injury.

A crucial difference among elite snowboarders is the relatively higher proportion of knee injuries and fewer wrist injuries [18].

Among elite snowboarders, the most common injury type was knee injuries, followed by the head, both being more frequent in the jumping disciplines, snowboard cross and halfpipe, compared to parallel giant slalom/parallel slalom. No differences between male and female snowboarders were found [15].

Understanding the specific injury mechanisms in snowboarding is crucial for implementing effective preventive measures and promoting safety within the sport.

Wrist injuries occur when snowboarders, who typically do not carry poles, attempt to break their falls using an open hand, putting their wrists at risk.

Lower-extremity injuries are less prevalent, but when they occur, the leading leg is more frequently affected than the trailing leg [24]. The underlying reasons for this phenomenon remain unclear and necessitate further investigation. Notably, the snowboarder's ankle, a unique injury specific to snowboarding, involves a fracture to the lateral process of the talus. This injury is believed to result from a combination of compression, forced inversion, or dorsiflexion, often experienced during jump landings. It is crucial to be cautious when diagnosing a snowboarder's ankle, as it can be misdiagnosed as a severe ankle sprain, potentially leading to inadequate treatment and long-term complications [25].

Unlike skiing, snowboarding has a lower incidence of knee ligament tears, mainly ACL tears. The lower knee injury rate in snowboarding compared to skiers difference is likely attributed to the no releasable binding system used in snowboarding, which prevents the application of valgus stress on one leg, a common mechanism for ACL tears in skiers. ACL tears in snowboarding predominantly occur among expert riders during improper landings from large jumps, known as flat landings. In this situation, the force is directed vertically through the leg and combines quadriceps contraction, low hamstring activation, and flexed knee; the ACL can be strained and torn. Additionally, ACL tears can occur when only one foot is attached to the snowboard, such as during chairlift loading or traversing flat areas [20].

The mechanics of snowboarding, involving the likelihood of falling backwards, increase the risk of spinal and potential head trauma. Jump-landing failure is the most common mechanism for spinal fracture except for snowboard cross, where collisions predominate.

Chronic injuries, such as tendonitis, can significantly impact a snowboarder's performance and overall enjoyment of the sport. In snowboarding, tendonitis commonly affects areas like the wrist, elbow, or knee due to repetitive motions and strain on these joints [26].

12.4 Diagnosis

Accurate and timely diagnosis of snowboarding-related injuries is paramount for appropriate treatment planning and optimal patient outcomes. In recent years, advancements in imaging modalities have significantly improved the diagnostic capabilities in this field.

X-ray imaging is widely used as an initial diagnostic tool for evaluating acute osteoarticular snowboarding injuries. It offers a fast and cost-effective way to assess skeletal structures and detect fractures, dislocations, and joint abnormalities. X-rays are beneficial for assessing snowboarding-related fractures of the extremities, such as wrist and ankle fractures. However, X-rays have limitations in visualizing soft tissue injuries and may miss subtle fractures, like scaphoid fractures, which can be radiographically occult in up to 25% of patients [27].

CT imaging is crucial in diagnosing complex fractures and spinal injuries and evaluating head, neck, and torso injuries in snowboarding accidents. CT offers detailed cross-sectional images that enhance the visualization of bony structures, allowing for accurate assessment of fracture patterns and joint involvement. With its speed and high spatial resolution, CT is valuable in identifying intra-articular fractures, evaluating joint dislocations, and assessing associated injuries such as internal organ damage or haemorrhage. For example, CT is the primary method in evaluating pelvic injuries following snowboarding trauma because it allows a better depiction and characterization of the true extent of pelvic fractures and potential associated soft tissue injuries. Furthermore, CT angiography became essential to detect active bleeding that might need urgent embolization if the patient was hemodynamically unstable [28]. CT is also the imaging modality of choice for the initial assessment of traumatic brain injuries. However, it is limited in evaluating the total extent of brain damage because it is insensitive to depicting diffuse axonal injury [29]. However, CT involves exposure to ionizing radiation, limiting its repeated use, particularly in paediatric populations.

Ultrasound imaging is a valuable tool for diagnosing snowboarding injuries, particularly for assessing soft tissue structures, joints, and superficial injuries. It is a safe, portable, non-invasive imaging modality and provides real-time imaging guidance during interventions such as joint aspirations or injections. Ultrasound effectively diagnoses tendon injuries, muscle strains, and joint effusions and identifies superficial soft tissue hematomas. However, ultrasound has operator-dependent limitations and may not penetrate deeper structures effectively, making it less suitable for evaluating more profound joint or spinal injuries.

MRI is an essential imaging modality for evaluating soft tissue injuries commonly associated with snowboarding accidents. It offers exceptional visualization of ligaments, tendons, muscles, and other soft tissue structures. MRI is invaluable in diagnosing injuries such as anterior cruciate ligament (ACL) tears, meniscal tears, rotator cuff tears, and labral injuries. Additionally, MRI can aid in identifying bone marrow oedema, assessing cartilage integrity, and detecting occult fractures. For example, in the case of shoulder dislocation, MRI should be performed to identify the type and extent of soft tissue damage and help with preoperative planning [30]. The non-invasive nature of MRI and its multiplanar imaging capabilities make it an excellent choice for the comprehensive evaluation of complex snowboarding injuries. However, MRI is relatively expensive and time-consuming, and it may not be suitable for patients with certain metallic implants or severe claustrophobia. MR arthrography was shown to be superior in identifying labral, cartilage, and partial-thickness rotator cuff tears but should be reserved under challenging specific cases [31].

Imaging modalities, including X-ray, CT, MRI, and ultrasound, play a pivotal role in diagnosing snowboarding-related injuries. Each modality has its strengths and limitations, and the choice of imaging technique depends on the suspected injury, clinical presentation, and availability of resources. A multimodal approach is necessary for a comprehensive evaluation, accurate diagnosis, and subsequent management of snowboarding injuries.

12.5 Treatment Options

Due to its high intensity and recklessness, snowboarding carries a high risk of injuries, which are becoming more common in orthopaedic practice due to increased participation.

When a snowboarding injury occurs, immediate care minimizes further damage and promotes recovery. The primary goal is stabilizing the injured person and ensuring their safety; this includes immobilizing suspected fractures, controlling bleeding, and keeping the injured individual warm. A ski patrol team trained in emergency response is present in competitions and most ski resorts.

Medical assistance is crucial in nearby terrain parks, which account for 20% of snowboarding injuries [32].

Assistance on basic first aid knowledge, including CPR and the ability to manage head and neck injuries, must be provided by personnel. These professionals are equipped to handle snowboarding injuries on the slopes. Ski patrol members assess the situation, provide first aid, and transport the injured person to the appropriate medical facility. Their expertise and timely intervention can significantly impact the outcome of an injury.

Following the initial assessment, diagnostic imaging techniques may be employed to evaluate the extent of the injury. An accurate diagnosis is crucial for determining the appropriate course of treatment.

The PRICE (Protection, Rest, Ice, Compression, Elevation) [33] method is often the first-line treatment for many snowboarding injuries. Rest allows the body time to heal, while ice reduces swelling and inflammation. Compression through bandages or braces supports the injured area, and elevation helps minimize swelling.

Physical therapy may be recommended for less severe injuries to regain strength, flexibility, and range of motion. Therapeutic exercises, stretches, and modalities such as heat or cold therapy aid in the recovery process.

Also utilized are medications like non-steroidal anti-inflammatory drugs (NSAIDs) that can help alleviate pain and reduce inflammation associated with snowboarding injuries.

In cases where snowboarding injuries are severe or complex or fail to respond to non-surgical treatments, surgery may be required. Surgical procedures commonly required to treat snowboarders include fracture fixation, ligament reconstruction, and joint repair. Orthopaedic surgeons can utilize advanced techniques like arthroscopy to minimize invasiveness and promote faster recovery.

In the case of fractures and dislocations, immobilization is essential, using splints, casts, or braces to allow the bones to heal correctly. In some cases, surgical intervention may be necessary to realign the bones and fix fractures with pins, screws, or plates.

The PRICE method is the initial step for treating sprains and strains. Rehabilitation exercises, stretching, and strengthening activities are essential for restoring the affected area's mobility, flexibility, and strength.

In ligament tears, conservative treatment can be managed for partial tears or minor ligament injuries, including rest, physical therapy, and knee braces with spontaneous healing without any interventions [34]. Complete tears or severe ligament injuries may require surgical reconstruction, where the damaged ligament is replaced or repaired using grafts or sutures.

After a concussion, it is essential to rest physically and mentally, allowing the brain to recover. Close monitoring for symptoms and an evaluation by a healthcare professional are essential to assess the severity of the concussion and provide appropriate guidance for recovery.

Suspected spinal injuries require immediate immobilization using a rigid collar or spinal board to prevent further damage. Ski patrol or medical professionals should handle spinal injuries with extreme care, and immediate transportation to a medical facility equipped to handle spinal injuries is crucial for proper evaluation, diagnosis, and treatment.

Overuse injuries (e.g. tendonitis) often improve with rest from the aggravating activity and modifying the snowboarding technique or equipment.

Exercises, manual therapy, and stretches reduce pain, improve flexibility, and strengthen the affected area, especially when introducing a slow progressive loading programme [35].

12.6 Return to Performance

Returning to snowboarding after an injury is a challenging process. It requires careful consideration, preparation, and a gradual approach to ensure a safe return.

Before resuming snowboarding, obtaining medical clearance from a healthcare professional is crucial, ensuring that the injury has adequately healed and that the body is ready to withstand the physical demands of snowboarding.

Completing the prescribed rehabilitation program is essential for restoring strength, flexibility, and functional abilities. Physical therapists are crucial in guiding rehabilitation, gradually reintroducing sport-specific exercises, and monitoring progress.

Gradually increasing resistance using weights, resistance bands, or bodyweight exercises helps rebuild muscle strength and endurance.

Neuromuscular control exercises focus on improving balance, proprioception, and coordination [36]. Utilizing balance boards, stability balls, or foam pads can challenge the body's stability and enhance control over movements, reducing the risk of re-injury and incorporating exercises that target the core muscles. Exercises that mimic snowboarding movements help re-establish the neuromuscular patterns required for the sport.

Functional training and sport-specific exercises are essential to regain snowboarding skills and readiness.

These activities focus on mimicking the movements and demands of snowboarding; this can also include practicing stance adjustments, edge transitions, and body positioning on dry land or in controlled snowboarding environments.

Therapists can tailor exercises to target the injured muscles and joints. Slowly reintroducing snowboarding practice in a controlled manner allows the body to adapt to the demands of the sport [37]. Start with gentle terrain, and progress to more challenging slopes, gradually incorporating different manoeuvres, turns, and tricks.

Implementing a well-structured training plan with periodization and progression is essential for optimizing rehabilitation and return to sport.

Periodization divides the training into specific phases to help manage intensity, volume, and recovery. These phases can include an initial rehabilitation phase, a strength and conditioning phase, and a specific snowboarding skill development phase.

Increasing the difficulty and intensity of exercises and snowboarding activities ensures a safe and gradual return. Progression should be individualized based on the injury, physical capabilities, and guidance from medical professionals or trainers.

Regular monitoring of progress, pain levels, and any signs of overuse or re-injury is crucial. Adjustments to the training plan may be necessary to address any setbacks or plateaus.

Returning to snowboarding after an injury can be mentally challenging. Building confidence and trust in the injured body part is crucial. It can be achieved through positive self-talk, visualization techniques, and gradually exposing oneself to progressively challenging snowboarding situations. Mental preparation involves setting realistic goals, managing expectations, and maintaining a positive mindset. Working with a sports psychologist or mental skills coach can be beneficial in developing coping strategies, enhancing focus, and dealing with any lingering fear or anxiety related to the injury.

Snowboarding skills may need refinement after a prolonged period of recovery. General rules for return after injuries include a fully functional range of motion and strength so that athletes can protect themselves and minimize additional risk [32].

Athletes involved in adventure/extreme sports usually return to active practice even after life-threatening or disabling injuries [13].

However, returning to snowboarding after an injury requires a systematic and patient approach. The key elements to consider are physical and psychological readiness, proper planning, and injury prevention strategies. By following a well-structured return-to-sport plan and prioritizing safety, snowboarders can enjoy their favourite sport again while minimizing the risk of future injuries.

12.7 Prevention

The primary prevention of injury among snowboarders enthusiasts may ultimately have a tremendous public health impact in reducing the burden of injuries and their chronic consequences (e.g. abandonment of sports, immobility, and obesity) [38].

Injury prevention is of the utmost importance in advanced and elite snowboarding to ensure a safe activity on slopes and pipes. Collaboration with professionals on the ski slopes, medical experts, and event planners is crucial for injury prevention. Their involvement ensures proper course design, monitoring of slope conditions, and prompt medical assistance if needed.

Injury prevention in snowboarding requires a comprehensive approach encompassing physical preparation, proper equipment, terrain awareness, and collaboration with professionals. By prioritizing physical training, flexibility, a proper progression to more demanding freestyle tricks, and appropriate gear, snowboarders can reduce the risk of injuries and enjoy a safe and fulfilling experience on the slopes.

12.7.1 Training

12.7.1.1 Physical Training

Maintaining proper physical fitness by applying regular conditioning and strength training exercises is fundamental to improving their overall strength, endurance, and stability. Also, skill level and experience are essential for injury prevention [39]. Focus on exercises that target core muscles, leg strength, and balance, as these areas are vital for maintaining control and stability while snowboarding [40]. Screening methods that assess neuromuscular control, such as jumping tests, can help predict the risk of injuries [41].

Adequate flexibility is essential to prevent muscle strains and injuries by incorporating regular stretching routines to improve hip, hamstrings, quadriceps, and upper body flexibility. Additionally, warming up before hitting the slopes with dynamic exercises, such as jogging or light aerobic activities, helps increase blood flow, warm the muscles, and reduce the risk of injury.

12.7.2 Trick Progression in Elite Freestyle Snowboarding

In freestyle tricks, progression is usually achieved intermittently, moving through different stages over the course of the year, also depending on the availability of suitable environmental conditions, and training facilities, balancing the time devoted to progression with that allocated to consolidation, competition periods, and rehabilitation from injuries.

Willmott and Collins described the pathway for trick development from the initial thought process and visualization to the use of supporting training modalities (including trampolines and airbags) to on-snow training.

Cognitive skills are a crucial and necessary part of skill acquisition and involve visual and kinaesthetic imagery.

Concerning supporting training modalities, athletes indicated using training methods, including a trampoline for general aerial awareness and airbags (providing a cushioned landing) for specific preparation.

Once athletes have landed on their feet 3 or 4 times in a row, they are ready to progress to snow [38].

Some athletes find that soft snow conditions at summer training camps and in the springtime are more conducive to introducing new tricks on the snow.

The duration of trick development considerably varies (from days to months or even years) within and between participants [42].

12.7.3 Equipment

Proper equipment is essential for safety in snowboarding.

More recent research supports the protective value of helmets in reducing the risk of head injuries without increasing the risk of neck injuries among skiers and snowboarders, despite some authors' fears that helmets may increase the number of injuries to the neck [43]. Choosing a helmet specifically for snowboarding with appropriate safety certifications ensures a snug and secure fit.

Snowboarders should consider wearing wrist guards to help prevent wrist fractures and sprains, the most common injuries in snowboarding [44]. Impact-resistant clothing, such as padded jackets and pants, can protect against bumps, falls, and impacts with obstacles.

Regularly inspecting and maintaining bindings and boots is crucial for proper functionality and safety. Ensure that bindings are securely fastened and boots fit correctly to provide optimal support and control. *Artificial intelligence tools (ChatGPT, OpenAI; Grammarly Inc.) were used exclusively for English language revision and editorial assistance. No AI tools were used for data analysis, interpretation, or generation of scientific content.*

References

1. Skicanada. What is snowboarding https://www.skicanada.org/ready/what-is-snowboarding/. Accessed on 14 June 2023 (n.d.)
2. Freethepowder.com. History of snowboard. https://www.freethepowder.com/pages/history-of-snowboarding. Accessed on 14 June 2023 (n.d.)
3. Olympics.com. History of snowboard. https://olympics.com/en/sports/snowboard/. Accessed on 14 June 2023 (n.d.)
4. Britannicas.com. (Bright, Torah) snowboarding https://www.britannica.com/sports/snowboarding. Accessed on 14 June 2023 (n.d.)
5. World Snowboard Federation. History. https://www.worldsnowboardfederation.org/. Accessed on 14 June 2023 (n.d.)
6. Funsporting.com. Top Snowboarding Competitions You Need to Know. https://funsporting.com/top-snowboarding-competitions-you-need-to-know/. Accessed on 14 June 2023 (n.d.)
7. Olympics.com. Shaun White. https://olympics.com/en/athletes/shaun-white. Accessed on 16 June 2023 (n.d.)
8. Olympics.com. Chloe Kim. https://olympics.com/it/atleti/chloe-kim. Accessed on 16 June 2023 (n.d.)
9. Freerideworldtour.com. Snowboard legend Terje Haakonsen to compete in Japan. https://www.freerideworldtour.com/news/snowboard-legend-terje-haakonsen-compete-japan. Accessed on 16 June 2023 (n.d.)
10. Dope magazine (Morgan, Daniel). Snowboard's trick. Retrieved on June 17, 2023 from https://www.dopesnow.com/it/mag/trick-snowboard-nomi/#butter-tricks (n.d.)
11. Rinding boards. A guide to freestyle snowboarding. Retrieved on June 17, 2023 from https://www.ridingboards.com/freestyle-snowboarding/ (n.d.)
12. Academic.com. List of snowboard tricks. Retrieved on June 17, 2023 from https://en.everybodywiki.com/List_of_snowboard_tricks.+ (n.d.)
13. Feletti F, Brymer E. Injury in kite buggying: the role of the 'out-of-buggy experience'. J Orthop Surg Res. 2018;13(1):104. https://doi.org/10.1186/s13018-018-0818-x.
14. Stenroos A, Handolin L. Incidence of recreational alpine skiing and snowboarding injuries: six years experience in the largest ski resort in Finland. Scand J Surg. 2015;104(2):127–31. https://doi.org/10.1177/1457496914532249.
15. Major DH, Steenstrup SE, Bere T, Bahr R, Nordsletten L. Injury rate and injury pattern among elite world

cup snowboarders: a 6-year cohort study. Br J Sports Med. 2014;48(1):18–22. https://doi.org/10.1136/bjsports-2013-092573.
16. Reynier V, Soulé B, Pabion-Mouriès J. Snowpark users' multi-faceted relationship with risk. Eur J Sport Soc. 2022;20(2):118–39. https://doi.org/10.1080/16138171.2022.2032919.
17. Feletti F, Brymer E. Pediatric and adolescent injury in skateboarding. Res Sports Med. 2018;26(sup1):129–49. https://doi.org/10.1080/15438627.2018.1438285.
18. Seleznev A, Shah NV, Desai R, Le C, Cleary P, Naziri Q, et al. Trends of snowboarding-related fractures that presented to emergency departments in the United States, 2010 to 2016. Ann Transl Med. 2018;6(11):200.
19. Owens BD, Nacca C, Harris AP, Feller RJ. Comprehensive review of skiing and snowboarding injuries. J Am Acad Orthop Surg. 2018;26(1):e1–10.
20. Telgheder ZL, Kistler BJ. Ski and snowboard – related orthopedic injuries. Orthop Clin North Am. 2020;51(4):461–9. https://doi.org/10.1016/j.ocl.2020.06.004.
21. Bianchi G, Brugger O, Niemann S. Skiing and snowboarding in Switzerland: trends in injury and fatality rates over time. In: Scher I, Greenwald R, Petrone N, editors. Snow sports trauma and safety. Cham: Springer Open; 2017. p. 29–39.
22. Bigdon SF, Gewiess J, Hoppe S, Exadaktylos AK, Benneker LM, Fairhurst PG, et al. Spinal injury in alpine winter sports: a review. Scand J Trauma Resusc Emerg Med. 2019;27(1):1–11.
23. De Roulet A, Inaba K, Strumwasser A, Chouliaras K, Lam L, Benjamin E, et al. Severe injuries associated with skiing and snowboarding: a national trauma data bank study. J Trauma Acute Care Surg. 2017;82(4):781–6.
24. Wijdicks CA, et al. Injuries in elite and recreational snowboarders. Br J Sports Med. 2014;48(1):11–7.
25. Kim S, et al. Snowboarding injuries: trends over time and comparisons with alpine skiing injuries. Am J Sports Med. 2012;40(4):770–6.
26. Feletti F, editor. Extreme sports medicine. Cham: Springer; 2017. https://doi.org/10.1007/978-3-319-28265-7.
27. Jenkins PJ, Slade K, Huntley JS, Robinson CM. A comparative analysis of the accuracy, diagnostic uncertainty and cost of imaging modalities in suspected scaphoid fractures. Injury. 2008;39(07):768–74.
28. Feletti F. Sports radiology: A key driver of clinical decision-making. Diagnostics (Basel). 2025;15(15):1977. https://doi.org/10.3390/diagnostics15151977.
29. Davis PC. Expert panel on neurologic imaging. Head trauma. AJNR Am J Neuroradiol. 2007;28(08):1619–21.
30. Bohyn C, Flores DV, Murray T, Mohr B, Cresswell M. Imaging review of snowboard injuries. Semin Musculoskelet Radiol. 2022;26(1):54–68.
31. Amini B, Beckmann NM, Beaman FD, et al. Expert panel on musculoskeletal imaging. ACR appropriateness criteria® shoulder pain-traumatic. J Am Coll Radiol. 2018;15(5S):S171–88.
32. Helmig K, Treme G, Richter D. Management of injuries in snowboarders: rehabilitation and return to activity. Open Access J Sport Med. 2018;9:221–31.
33. Bleakley CM, Taylor JB, Dischiavi SL, Doherty C, Delahunt E. Rehabilitation exercises reduce re-injury post ankle sprain, but the content and parameters of an optimal exercise program have yet to be established: a systematic review and meta-analysis. Arch Phys Med Rehabil. 2019;100(7):1367–75. https://doi.org/10.1016/j.apmr.2018.10.005.
34. Razi M, Soufali AP, Ziabari EZ, Dadgostar H, Askari A, Arasteh P. Treatment of concomitant ACL and MCL injuries: spontaneous healing of complete ACL and MCL tears. J Knee Surg. 2021;34(12):1329–36.
35. Cardoso TB, Pizzari T, Kinsella R, Hope D, Cook JL. Current trends in tendinopathy management. Best Pract Res Clin Rheumatol. 2019;33(1):122–40. https://doi.org/10.1016/j.berh.2019.02.001.
36. Zemková E, Kováčiková Z. Sport-specific training induced adaptations in postural control and their relationship with athletic performance. Front Hum Neurosci. 2023;16:1007804.
37. Kuepper T, Huber N, Netzer N, Schoeffl V. Rehabilitation and recovery training after snowboard accidents. Med Sport. 2009;13(1):1–4.
38. Emery CA, Pasanen K. Current trends in sport injury prevention. Best Pract Res Clin Rheumatol. 2019; https://doi.org/10.1016/j.berh.2019.02.009.
39. McKenna J, Hammond C. Perspectives on injuries in snow- boarders. J R Soc Promot Heal. 2007;127(4):181–9.
40. McGill S. Core training: evidence translating to better performance and injury prevention. Strength Cond J. 2010;32(3):33–46.
41. Hewett TE, Myer GD, Ford KR, et al. Biomechanical measures of neuromuscular control and valgus loading of the knee predict anterior cruciate ligament injury risk in female athletes: a prospective study. Am J Sports Med. 2005;33(4):492–501.
42. Willmott T, Collins D. A retrospective analysis of trick progression in elite Freeskiing and snowboarding. Int Sport Coaching J. 2017;4:1–12. https://doi.org/10.1123/iscj.2016-0003.
43. Hébert-Losier K, Holmberg HC. What are the exercise-based injury prevention recommendations for recreational alpine skiing and snowboarding?: a systematic review. Sport Med. 2013;43(5):355–66.
44. Russell K, Hagel B, Francescutti LH. The effect of wrist guards on wrist and arm injuries among snowboarders: a systematic review. Clin J Sport Med. 2007;17(2):145–50. https://doi.org/10.1097/JSM.0b013e31803f901b.

13 Skydiving

Francesco Feletti, Benedetta Rossini,
Lucia Battara, and Aldo Carnevale

13.1 Introduction

According to the United States Parachute Association (USPA), approximately 4 million skydives were made in 2022 at 230 different drop zones, and the USPA currently lists a membership of more than 42,000 [1]. The number of recreational and sports skydiving participants slowly but constantly increases over time [1]. A parachute can be defined as an aerodynamic decelerator [2]. Skydiving, also called parachuting, involves using a parachute for recreational or competitive purposes to slow a diver's descent to the ground after jumping from an aeroplane or another high place [2]. Skydiving has come a long way since the beginning of parachuting, which dates back to 1100 in China, where shortly after the invention of the umbrella, there were attempts to use it as a rigid parachute [3]. An anonymous manuscript dating back to the 1470s reports the oldest parachute design: a free-hanging man grabbing a crossbar frame connected to a conical canopy [3]. Shortly after, around 1485, the sketch of a more sophisticated parachute appeared in the Codex Atlanticus by Leonardo da Vinci [3]. Among the first experimental applications were the launches of the Frenchman Lenormand, who launched himself in 1732 from the Montpellier Observatory, and above all that of the Frenchman André-Jacques Garnerin, who in 1797 jumped from a hot air balloon [2].

Further experience led parachutes to become more compact and versatile.

In the second half of the nineteenth century, in the western United States, Park Van Tassel and Thomas Scott Baldwin, two aerial exhibitionists and balloonists, introduced new methods of parachute jumping from balloons, promoted ballooning and parachuting internationally and introduced women to these sports [4].

In 1911, Grant Morton made the first parachute jump from an aeroplane, a Wright Model B, at Venice Beach, California. In the same year, Gleb Kotelnikov invented the first knapsack parachute, folded into a pack to be worn on the back and pulled out by a line, later popularized by Paul Letterman and Kathchen Paulus.

F. Feletti (✉) · B. Rossini
Dipartimento di Medicina Traslazionale e per la Romagna, Università di Ferrara, Ferrara, Italy

Unità Operativa di Radiologia, Ospedale S. Maria delle Croci, Ausl della Romagna, Ravenna, Italy

EXTREMESPORTMED, International Society of Medicine for Outdoor Physical Activity and Extreme Sports, Città Metropolitana di Bologna, Bologna, Italy
e-mail: francesco.feletti@unife.it; benedetta.rossini@edu.unife.it

L. Battara · A. Carnevale
Dipartimento di Medicina Traslazionale e per la Romagna, Università di Ferrara, Ferrara, Italy

Unità Operativa di Radiologia, Arcispedale S. Anna, Aosp Ferrara, Cona, Ferrara, Italy
e-mail: aldo.carnevale@unife.it

H. Jones, A. Lukaszenko (eds.), *Injury Prevention and Care in Artistic Sports*,
https://doi.org/10.1007/978-3-032-18105-3_13

The first military use of the parachute was in World War I by artillery observers on tethered observation balloons [5]. In the 1920s and 1930s, numerous studies and experiences led to the creation of effective and safe parachutes, to the extent that during World War II, parachutes were used not only as a rescue system but also for launching units in combat zones.

The first world parachuting championships were held in Yugoslavia in 1951, followed by subsequent world championships under the auspices of the Fédération Aéronautique Internationale (FAI) [2].

FAI, also known as the World Air Sports Federation, was founded in 1905. It is a non-governmental and non-profit international organization aiming to further aeronautical and astronautical activities worldwide. The FAI is currently recognized by the International Olympic Committee (IOC); it ratifies skydiving world and continental records and coordinates the organization of international skydiving competitions [6].

The FAI Skydiving Commission (ISC) oversees FAI's parachuting and indoor skydiving activities, including World Records and International Competitions.

While skydiving is not an Olympic sport, it has been included in the sports program of the World Games since 1997.

A skydiver's equipment comprises one primary and one reserve parachute packed into a specialized backpack with a chest strap and leg straps cinched to keep the jumper securely fastened [6]. Skydiving equipment has advanced considerably over the last several years, focusing on enhancing safety, performance, and user experience. Key advancements include:

- Improvements in parachute designs.
- The development of more reliable and efficient canopies.
- The introduction of Automatic Activation Devices (AADs) for enhanced safety.
- The evolution of harness and container systems for better fit and functionality.

Altimeters have become more accurate and feature rich, helmets have improved in design and safety features, and skydiving suits have seen advancements in design and materials.

Additionally, the availability of advanced training tools and equipment has improved safety in the sport.

13.1.1 Disciplines

In skydiving, several disciplines are recognized by the FAI ISC [6].

13.1.1.1 The Classics

The two oldest skydiving disciplines are freefall style and accuracy landing, also called the classic.

In freefall style, control and correctness of the execution of a prescribed sequence of manoeuvres are judged from a video recording captured by a ground-based camera. Accuracy landing involves landing as close as possible to the centre of a target.

13.1.1.2 Artistic Events

In the early nineties, some skydivers tested manoeuvres derived from acrobatics and ice skating while others tried jumping with snowboards (sky surfing). Both activities catalysed media attention, and the World Freestyle Federation organized championships.

Through the work of a specific committee, which today is named "Artistic Events", the FAI Parachuting Commission (IPC) incorporated freestyle in the form of free-flying, the only discipline that incorporates all dimensional axes during the freefall part of a parachute jump.

On the contrary, skysurfing on a competition scale was retired. Artistic Events consist of obligatory (see https://www.fai.org/news/video-animations-line-artistic-compulsory-sequence) and free routines performed during seven skydives. Teams consist of one or two athletes and a camera flyer that captures the images for judging the performances.

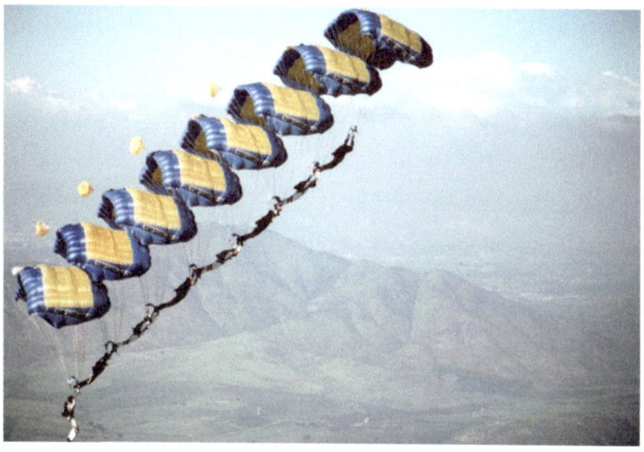

Fig. 13.1 Eight members of the "Leapfrogs," the Navy's parachute team, descend in a stacked-canopy formation (Photo by Melinda Larson, San Diego, California)

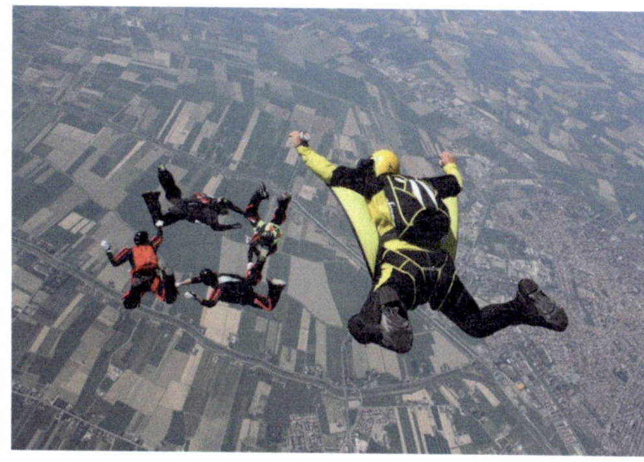

Fig. 13.2 Four-way formation skydiving. One team member wears a camera and films the video to be judged. (Photo courtesy Dario Vecchiato; Ravenna, Italy)

13.1.1.3 Canopy Formation

In Canopy formation, teams of two (two-way) or four (four-way) skydivers create different figures under open canopies. The team's videographer produces the video that the judges evaluate immediately after landing (Fig. 13.1).

13.1.1.4 Canopy Piloting

Canopy piloting is a fairly new, high-speed discipline that involves small and very agile parachutes and is practiced over a stretch of water for safety reasons and to allow bystanders to watch the stunts from a short distance. Athletes accelerate their parachutes through steep turns and then plan over the water's surface to enter the course. There are three traditional specialties:

Accuracy involves navigating the water section close to the centre of a target.
Speed consists of flying the course in the shortest time.
Distance involves flying the maximum distance.

In recent years, a new subdiscipline that shows artistic elements, freestyle, has increased popularity. In freestyle, the skydivers perform tricks with their bodies and parachute while dragging the water. A panel of judges score the trick's difficulty, proficiency in the execution, and artistic style.

13.1.1.5 Formation Skydiving

In formation skydiving, a team comprises four (four-way) or eight (eight-way) performers and one videographer (Fig. 13.2). Teams perform a designated sequence or series of formations drawn from an international pool.

The discipline can be practiced in the prone position (with a belly to earth) or vertically (with either feet or head toward the ground).

Judging is based on the videographer's footage of each round, and technical performance is assessed.

13.1.1.6 Indoor Skydiving

Over the last two decades, indoor skydiving tunnels have opened in cities worldwide, creating a boom, especially in the last 7 years.

The tunnels are circular spaces of varying diameters in which electric motors produce a strong vertical airflow; skydiving evolutions can be watched through the tunnel's transparent vertical walls. The public can watch the flyers revolve and rotate inside the tunnel, with the added value of the competition being easily visible to spectators.

Competitions consist of two different events: *indoor formation skydiving* and *artistic events*.

Indoor formation skydiving consists of a team of four participants executing a series of predefined compulsory formations.

Artistic events consist of *solo freestyle* and *dynamic flying*.

Solo freestyle is a solo discipline where the athletes perform compulsory and free routines. The competitor can choose to fly the free routine to music.

Dynamic flying was created in 2012; it involves flying in 3D, using all the space of a vertical wind tunnel.

It is practised in teams of four flyers (D4W) or two flyers (D2W) and in two subdisciplines: *speed round* and *free round*. In the *speed round*, skydivers must complete a series of synchronized compulsory patterns faster.

Free round is a judged competition where technical and artistic aspects are assessed during a set of creative evolution freely proposed by each team.

13.1.1.7 Parachute-Ski

It is a discipline recognized by the ISC that derives from a combination of skiing and skydiving; in competitions, the athlete performs an accuracy landing onto a slope followed by a Giant Slalom on the skis.

13.1.1.8 Speed Skydiving

In speed skydiving, the aim is to achieve and maintain the highest possible terminal velocity. Thanks to the minimization of drag by streamlining the body, generally in a head-down position, it is possible to achieve 530 km/h (330 mph) speeds, which are more than double the terminal velocity in the traditional belly-to-earth position (200 km/h) [6].

High-altitude jumps, thanks to the reduced air pressure even, may require the support of supplemental oxygen, allowing an increased freefall speed of far more than 1000 km/h, with the top speed record of 1357 km/h (843 mph) obtained by Felix Baumgartner with the Red Bull Stratos jump.

13.1.1.9 Wingsuit Flying

In 2015, FAI officially recognized wingsuit performance flying and wingsuit acrobatics as competition formats.

In wingsuit performance flying, time, distance, and speed are measured over separate flying sessions using a GPS logging device within the competition window (3000 m to 2000 m AGL).

Wingsuit acrobatics involves a competition between two-way teams with a camera flyer, including compulsory moves from a dive pool and free rounds. The flying style is a crucial element in these competitions, and critical aspects are body position, smoothness of flying, controlled docks, and forward flying speed.

13.2 Art and Skydiving

Artistic elements in skydiving are prominently featured in disciplines such as freestyle and freefly. These disciplines combine creativity, technical skill, and choreography to create visually captivating performances in the sky. The aesthetics of body positioning, body lines, and symmetry play a crucial role in presenting a visually appealing routine. Athletes often incorporate visually striking costumes, colourful jumpsuits, or skydiving suit designs to enhance the visual impact of their performances.

Apart from the disciplines mentioned above, skydivers may express their artistic side in special stunts such as night jumps, big ways (large formation jumps) (Fig. 13.3), or stuff jumps, in which skydivers jump out with objects (Fig. 13.4).

Artistic elements catalyse the attention of social media, which have played an influential role in promoting skydiving, expanding its reach to a broader audience, connecting skydivers worldwide, and creating a platform for sharing the thrills. Also, including skydiving disciplines in major sporting events like X games and the Red Bull Air Race has brought skydiving to a large audience. On 14 October 2012, 8 million people went onto YouTube to witness the game-changing moment when Austrian skydiver Felix Baumgartner completed a parachute jump from 38,969.4 m, smashing eight world records. He became the first human to break the sound barrier in freefall, achieved the highest freefall parachute jump (38,969.4 m/127,852 ft), and attained the fastest speed in freefall (1,357.6 km/h/843.6 mph) [7]. Following this accomplishment, Felix Baumgartner became the star of the Red Bull

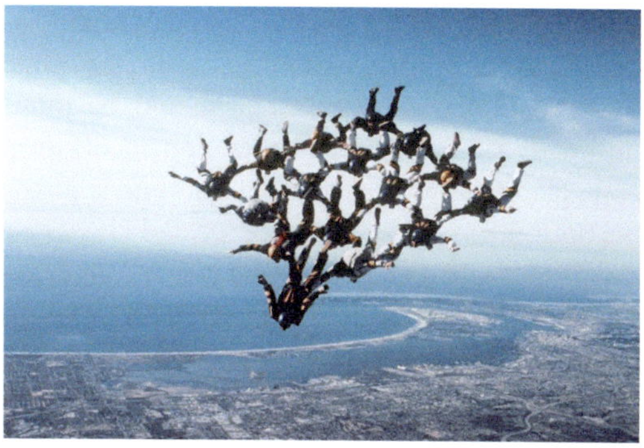

Fig. 13.3 Members of the "Leapfrogs," the Navy's parachute team, form a 16-man diamond formation during a free-fall descent. (Photo by Melinda Larson, San Diego, California)

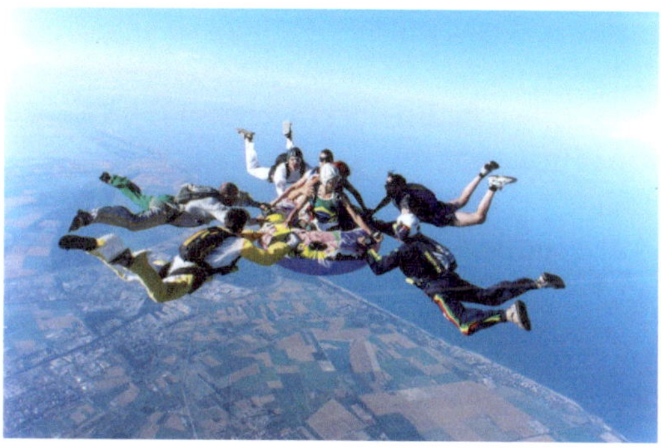

Fig. 13.4 Stuff jump with an inflatable dinghy. (Photo courtesy Dario Vecchiato, Ravenna, Italy)

commercial in 2012, and this media event played a significant role in promoting skydiving on a global scale. More recently, the American skydiver Luke Aikins made headlines in 2016 for completing a skydive without a parachute or wingsuit. He jumped from an altitude of 7,600 meters (25,000 feet) and landed in a net [8].

13.3 Epidemiology of More Frequent Injuries

In skydiving, potential injuries range from minor abrasions to life-threatening events. Existing data suggest that the incidence of fatal accidents has decreased over time. In the USA, the death rate was about 1.06 per 100,000 jumps during the period of 1993–1999 [9]. Between 1994 and 2003, 0.8 deaths were recorded in Sweden per 100,000 jumps [10]. From 2000 to 2004, the rate was 0.3 deaths per 100,000 jumps [11]. In a more recent French study conducted between 2010 and 2019, the death rate was 0.57 per 100,000 jumps, 0.54 per 100,000 jumps for student skydivers, and 0.63 per 100,000 jumps for experienced skydivers [12].

In freestyle and canopy piloting, high-speed canopy turns can create similar dangers to steep spirals in powered paragliding, particularly regarding high G-forces, reduced blood flow to the brain, and the risk of blackouts or loss of control [13].

The reported injury rates in the 1980s and 1990s varied from 120 to 360 injuries per 100,000 jumps [14–16]. During the 2000 and 2001 World Freefall Skydiving Conventions [17], the injury rate was 174/100,000 jumps, confirmed in Sweden by the data collected by Westman [18]. According to the data collected by the French Parachuting Federation (FFP), between 2010 and 2019, an overall injury rate of 49 injuries per 100,000 jumps was calculated. This data breakdown implicated 133 injuries per 100,000 jumps in the student group, 28 injuries per 100,000 jumps in the experienced group, and 51 injuries per 100,000 jumps in the tandem group [14].

Most of the reported injuries are to the lower-limb extremities (51%) followed by the upper arm (19%), the back (17.1–18%), the head/neck (7–8.6%), and the shoulder (5.7%) [17, 19]. Lower-limb injuries are frequent and are represented by fractures, sprains, and contusions affecting the leg, the ankle, and the foot. These injuries generally occur due to collision to the ground due to improper landing techniques or when the parachute fails to slow down descent sufficiently before touchdown. After a correct parachute opening, a typical nonfatal injury event is caused by gusts of wind or miscalculation (e.g. off headwind, low turn, incorrect horizontal levelling for landing), resulting in a violent landing leading to lower-limb and/or back injuries [18].

Back and spine injuries can happen during freefall and excessive deceleration during canopy deployment or landing. Sudden movements, improper body positioning, or a hard landing can contribute to strains, sprains, or more severe spinal injuries, including cervical spine fractures [20, 21].

Wrist and hand injuries, including fractures, sprains, or dislocations, often occur during landing to absorb the impact to the ground.

Skydiving stresses the shoulders, especially during parachute deployment [22]. Indoor skydiving, in particular, may increase the risk of anterior dislocations, as an already-abducted shoulder can be forcefully moved into hyper-external rotation [23].

Head and neck injuries are relatively uncommon in skydiving. These types of injuries typically occur in high-speed or impact-related incidents, ranging from concussions to more severe traumatic brain injuries. According to a study by T.F. Rooks, wing loading has been found to impact the resultant acceleration and angular rates experienced by the head and body, potentially contributing to the risk for parachute opening shock (POS)–induced neck pain [24].

During a skydive, in addition to acute traumas, there is also a potential for developing chronic clinical conditions. The human body undergoes trauma due to the forces and pressure differences experienced during this period. Minor strains, impacts, and micro-traumas that may not result in acute injuries can accumulate and lead to chronic conditions. Among these exposures, one of the most significant is the POS [25, 26]. During the POS, the parachute canopy suspends the skydiver from the shoulders. As the body is parallel to the ground during free fall, the skydiver is subjected to a force hyperextending all the vertebrae and neck. This event can result in a loss of stability in the muscles and spinal cord, particularly in the neck region, which may lead to trauma and injuries in the thoracic, lumbar, and especially the cervical vertebrae [26–28].

13.4 Diagnosis

Skydiving injuries require a multidisciplinary approach involving emergency medical personnel, radiologists, surgeons, and other healthcare professionals.

A keystone of trauma management is the so-called golden hour, stressing that the time between injury and treatment should be minimized. It is a crucial consideration in off-drop zone landings, where an initial lag time is possible until the skydiver has been located [18].

At the emergency department, a skydiving trauma may initially be considered a high-energy trauma, reasonably similar to a motorcycle crash, and critical care unit admission should be considered. Further transport to a trauma centre must be arranged if the patient's conditions exceed the local healthcare institution's assistance capabilities [18].

Skydivers at the scene can provide critical information about the trauma energy's speed, angles, and magnitude.

Electronic devices on the injured athlete should be preserved for later data analysis [17]. The first step in managing such injuries is the initial assessment of the trauma patient using a structured and systematic primary survey, like the airway, breathing, circulation, and disability (ABCD) survey of the trauma patient. Such an approach helps determine appropriate treatment strategies to maximize the chances of a successful recovery [29].

Following a skydiving incident, the first step is to perform a primary assessment of the injured individuals to ensure they are hemodynamically stable. A thorough physical examination is conducted to assess the extent and nature of the injuries. This examination may include checking for visible wounds, fractures, dislocations, soft tissue injuries, or any signs of internal bleeding or organ damage. Particular attention should be given to the spine, head, neck, and joints. Guidelines provide recommendations for immediate imaging in patients with suspected major haemorrhage and chest trauma and the use of whole-body CT for assessing patients with multiple injuries.

The high risk of lower-back injuries must be considered in skydivers.

Immediate imaging aims to identify active bleeding sites for appropriate haemorrhage control and to detect any other life-threatening conditions [30]. When skydiving is performed in remote or hostile environments, portable ultrasonography—potentially supported by telemedical guidance—may represent a valuable tool for the prompt diagnosis of life-threatening conditions, including cardiac tamponade and haemothorax, as well as to assist resuscitation manoeuvres and interventional procedures such as long-needle pericardiocentesis, chest tube placement in selected cases, or ultrasound-guided decompression of pneumothorax [31, 32].

For musculoskeletal injuries, imaging studies such as X-rays, computed tomography (CT) scans, or magnetic resonance imaging (MRI) may be performed. After the initial diagnosis, regular follow-up evaluations are essential to monitor the patient's progress, assess the healing process, and identify any complications [33].

13.5 Treatment Options

The specific treatment options for skydiving injuries can vary depending on the type and severity of the injury sustained.

In the event of fractures or dislocations, immobilization is typically the first step to prevent further damage. In more severe cases, surgical intervention may be necessary to realign the bones or joints.

Head and spinal injuries are potentially serious and require immediate medical attention [34]. Depending on the specific injury, treatment options may involve surgery, medication, immobilization, and rehabilitation.

The RICE method is commonly used to treat soft tissue injuries: rest, ice, compression, and elevation. Physical therapy may be recommended to restore strength and flexibility.

Superficial injuries like cuts, abrasions, and bruises can usually be managed with thorough cleaning, disinfection, and proper wound care. Stitches may be required for deep cuts or lacerations. Tetanus shots may also be administered if necessary.

13.6 Return to Performance

Physicians must consider that skydivers, as participants in many adventure and extreme sports [35–41], will likely return to their sport irrespective of their functional outcome. A poor outcome from nonoperative management will likely increase the risk of re-injury. They may also easily choose the surgical option when the physician proposes it as the solution, which more likely allows return to skydiving. At the same time, since skydivers may be obsessive about their sporting activities, they often display perfect adherence to rehabilitation.

Skydivers suffering from spinal injury and desiring to return to the sport require appropriate surgery and rehabilitation.

Rehabilitation should include retraining neck and back muscles due to the high force exposure related to parachute openings, which involve a deceleration estimated around 3–5G [18].

Joint stability is a crucial element in skydiving.

During landing, the ankle joint plays a fundamental role as skydivers, especially those flying fast parachutes, often run a few steps during landing, especially in no-wind conditions.

Therefore, a physiotherapist rehabilitating a skydiver with ankle trauma must clearly understand the speeds and angles in an uneventful or miscalculated landing.

In the case of a shoulder injury, a gradual return to skydiving may not be possible, as an "all-or-nothing" level of performance is required for the upper limbs.

Indeed, reserve parachute emergency procedures require bilateral hand and arm function; a shoulder joint dislocated mid-air can be life-threatening, mainly if the incapacitated hand is used for primary parachute activation. Moreover, a non-functioning arm can hinder an inexperienced skydiver from maintaining a stable body position during the free fall, with the following risk of entanglement at parachute deployment.

Therefore, beginners with shoulder problems and skydivers who have suffered shoulder injuries require relevant training, rehabilitation, and surgical stabilization whenever appropriate. Simulation in the vertical wind tunnel is possible for testing joint stability in a reduced-risk environment before a complete return.

Finally, in addition to muscular strength, endurance, and power, the proprioceptive component of rehabilitation must be integrated and progressed from an early stage of skydiver rehabilitation.

Specific exercises involve balance training, co-contraction, rhythmic stabilization, core stability, and plyometric exercises.

13.7 Prevention

Limited studies have analysed the effectiveness of various safety equipment, including helmet use, airbags, back guards, multichambered foams, or finger-tapping, in sports such as climbing, paragliding, skydiving, and base jumping [42, 43]. For instance, preventive ankle braces worn by military paratroopers have shown a reported injury reduction of 40–50% [44–46].

Jiang et al. demonstrated that knee braces provide protection on the sagittal plane for the hip, knee, and ankle and on the coronal plane only for the knee when used without the backpack. When used with the backpack, the knee brace still provides protection on the sagittal plane only for the knee and on the coronal plane for the knee, hip, and ankle [47].

Modern equipment in skydiving has decreased overall injuries and mortality. However, it has also increased injuries associated with high-speed landings [17]. Most injuries are caused by wing parachute piloting errors [19]. Therefore, to prevent skydiving injuries, providing adequate training on wing parachute piloting is crucial, both for novices and more experienced skydivers [19].

In conclusion, striking a balance between safety measures, the thrill of the activity, and the inherent risks is essential. While safety protocols are necessary to reduce injuries and fatalities, they may also be perceived as diminishing not only the appeal of the activity but also the artistic freedom of participants. By analysing sport-specific injury rates and patterns, both athletes and governing bodies can direct safety efforts where they will provide the greatest benefit to the community, without imposing unnecessary restrictions that could limit creativity and self-expression [48]. *AI tools (ChatGPT and Grammarly) were used for language editing and grammatical refinement.*

References

1. United States Parachute Association (USPA). https://www.uspa.org. Accessed on 3th July 2023
2. Turoff, MLH. "skydiving". Encyclopedia Britannica, 9 Aug. 2021. https://www.britannica.com/sports/skydiving. Accessed on 12 June 2023
3. White L. The invention of the parachute. Technol Cult. 1968;9(3):462–7.
4. Fogel GB. Sky rider: park Van tassel and the rise of ballooning in the west. University of New Mexico Press; 2021. p. 38–43.
5. Mahncke JOEO. Early Parachutes, an evaluation of the use of parachutes, with special emphasis on the Royal Flying Corps and the German Lufstreitkräfte, until 1918. South African Military History Journal (2000)
6. The Fédération Aéronautique Internationale, FAI. https://www.fai.org/federation. Accessed on 3 July 2023
7. Guinnes World Records. https://www.guinnessworldrecords.com/records/hall-of-fame/felix-baumgartner-first-person-to-break-sound-barrier-in-freefall. Accessed on 3 July 2023
8. Bisharat A. This Man Jumped Out of a Plane With No Parachute, https://www.nationalgeographic.com/adventure/article/skydiver-luke-aikins-freefalls-without-parachute. Accessed on 3 July 2023
9. Griffith JD, Hart CL. A summary of US skydiving fatalities: 1993–1999. Percept Mot Skills. 2002;94:1089–90. https://doi.org/10.2466/PMS.94.4.1089-1090.
10. Westman A, Björnstig U. Fatalities in Swedish skydiving. Accid Anal Prev. 2005;37(6):1040–8. https://doi.org/10.1016/j.aap.2005.06.002.
11. Hart CL, Griffith JD, Randell JA. An analysis of US parachuting fatalities: 2000–2004. Percept Mot Skills. 2006;103(3):896–900. https://doi.org/10.2466/PMS.103.3.896-900.
12. Fer C, Guiavarch M, Edouard P. Epidemiology of skydiving-related deaths and injuries: a 10-years prospective study of 6.2 million jumps between 2010 and 2019 in France. J Sci Med Sport. 2021;24(5):448–53.
13. Feletti F, Goin J. Accidents and injuries related to powered paragliding: a cross-sectional study. BMJ Open. 2014;4(8):e005508. https://doi.org/10.1136/bmjopen-2014-005508.
14. Amamilo SC, Samuel AW, Hesketh KT, et al. A prospective study of parachute injuries in civilians. The Journal of Bone and Joint Surgery. British volume. 1987;69(1):17–9.
15. Ellitsgaard N. Parachuting injuries: a study of 110,000 sports jumps. Br J Sports Med. 1987;21(1):13–7. https://doi.org/10.1136/bjsm.21.1.13.
16. Dawson M, Asghar M, Pryke S, et al. Civilian parachute injuries; 10 years on and no lessons learned. Injury. 1998;29(8):573–5. https://doi.org/10.1016/S0020-1383(97)00174-5.

17. Barrows TH, Mills TJ, Kassing SD. The epidemiology of skydiving injuries: world freefall convention, 2000–2001. J Emerg Med. 2005;28(1):63–8. https://doi.org/10.1016/j.jemermed.2004.07.008.
18. Westman A. Skydiving. In: Mei Dan O, Carmont MR, editors. Adventure and extreme sports injuries. London: Springer; 2013. p. 69–90.
19. Westman A, Björnstig U. Injuries in Swedish skydiving. Br J Sports Med. 2007;41(6):356–64. https://doi.org/10.1136/bjsm.2006.031682.
20. Flautt W, Rowland R, Westrick RB. Cervical fracture with posterior ligamentous injury while skydiving. J Orthop Sports Phys Ther. 2019;49(2):113. https://doi.org/10.2519/jospt.2019.8360.
21. Loebel F, Fekonja L, Vajkoczy P, Hecht N. Hangman's fracture caused by parachute opening deceleration captured on video. World Neurosurg. 2018;119:389–93. https://doi.org/10.1016/j.wneu.2018.08.089. Epub 2018 Aug 24
22. Westman A. Shoulder injuries have been noted as a recurring problem in skydiving. J Trauma. 2005;59(4):1033. https://doi.org/10.1097/01.ta.0000188014.44804.da.
23. Newcomb NL, Lester DR, Keyt LK, Zumsteg DM, Barry PA. Indoor skydiving: an emerging cause of anterior shoulder dislocations. Ochsner J. 2022;22(1):71–5. https://doi.org/10.31486/toj.21.0027.
24. Rooks TF, Novotny BL, McGovern SM, Winegar A, Shivers BL, Brozoski FT. Evaluation of head and body kinematics experienced during parachute opening shock. Mil Med. 2021;186(11–12):e1149–56.
25. Bar-Dayan Y, Weisbort M, Bar-Dayan Y, Velan GJ, Ravid M, Hendel D, Shemer J. Degenerative disease in lumbar spine of military parachuting instructors. J R Army Med Corps. 2003;149(4):260–4. https://doi.org/10.1136/jramc-149-04-03.
26. Coşkun Beyan A, Demiral Y, Dilek B, Alici NŞ, Bediz C, Çimrin A. Skydiving and the risk of cervical disc herniation. Int J Occup Med Environ Health. 2018;31(2):243–9. https://doi.org/10.13075/ijomeh.1896.01032.
27. Lo Martire R, Gladh K, Westman A, Lindholm P, Nilsson J, Äng BO. Neck muscle activity in skydivers during parachute opening shock. Scand J Med Sci Sports. 2016;26(3):307–16. https://doi.org/10.1111/sms.12428. Epub 2015 Mar 10
28. Gladh K, Lo Martire R, Äng BO, Lindholm P, Nilsson J, Westman A. Decelerations of parachute opening shock in skydivers. Aerosp Med Hum Perform. 2017;88(2):121–7. https://doi.org/10.3357/AMHP.4731.2017.
29. Galvagno SM Jr, Nahmias JT, Young DA. Advanced trauma life support® update 2019: management and applications for adults and special populations. Anesthesiol Clin. 2019;37(1):13–32. https://doi.org/10.1016/j.anclin.2018.09.009.
30. Glen J, Constanti M, Brohi K. Assessment and initial management of major trauma: summary of NICE guidance. BMJ. 2016;353:i3051. https://doi.org/10.1136/bmj.i3051.
31. Feletti F, Mucci V, Aliverti A. Chest ultrasonography in modern day extreme settings: from military setting and natural disasters to space flights and extreme sports. Can Respir J. 2018;2018:8739704. https://doi.org/10.1155/2018/8739704.
32. Pegoraro N, Rossini B, Giganti M, Brymer E, Monasterio E, Bouchat P, Feletti F. Telemedicine in sports under extreme conditions: data transmission, remote medical consultations, and diagnostic imaging. Int J Environ Res Public Health. 2023;20(14):6371. https://doi.org/10.3390/ijerph20146371.
33. Feletti F. Sports radiology: a key driver of clinical decision-making. Diagnostics (Basel). 2025;15(15):1977. https://doi.org/10.3390/diagnostics15151977.
34. Feletti F, editor. Extreme sports medicine. Cham: Springer; 2017. https://doi.org/10.1007/978-3-319-28265-7.
35. Feletti F, Brymer E. Injury in kite buggying: the role of the 'out-of-buggy experience'. J Orthop Surg Res. 2018;13(1):104. https://doi.org/10.1186/s13018-018-0818-x.
36. Feletti F, Brymer E. Pediatric and adolescent injury in skateboarding. Res Sports Med. 2018;26(sup1):129–49. https://doi.org/10.1080/15438627.2018.1438285.
37. Feletti F, Brymer E, Bonato M, Aliverti A. Injuries and illnesses related to dinghy-sailing on hydrofoiling boats. BMC Sports Sci Med Rehabil. 2021;13(1):118. https://doi.org/10.1186/s13102-021-00343-8.
38. Brymer E, Feletti F, Monasterio E, Schweitzer R. Editorial: understanding extreme sports: a psychological perspective. Front Psychol. 2020;10:3029. https://doi.org/10.3389/fpsyg.2019.03029.
39. Beer Y, Yona T, Arama Y, Lindner D, Garrigues G, Feletti F, Blond L, Gilat R. Kiteboarding injuries: epidemiology, common treatment strategies, and time to return to kiteboarding following injury. Clin J Sport Med. 2024;35(4):498–504. https://doi.org/10.1097/JSM.0000000000001270.
40. Feletti F, Saini G, Naldi S, Casadio C, Mellini L, Feliciani G, Zamprogno E. Injuries in medium to long-distance triathlon: a retrospective analysis of medical conditions treated in three editions of the ironman competition. J Sports Sci Med. 2022;21(1):58–67. https://doi.org/10.52082/jssm.2022.58.
41. Bouchat P, Feletti F, Monasterio E, Brymer E. What is so special about wingsuit BASE jumpers? A comparative study of their psychological characteristics. Int J Environ Res Public Health. 2022;19(5):3061. https://doi.org/10.3390/ijerph19053061.
42. Bigdon SF, Hecht V, Fairhurst PG, Deml MC, Exadaktylos AK, Albers CE. Injuries in alpine summer sports – types, frequency and prevention: a systematic review. BMC Sports Sci Med Rehabil. 2022;14(1):79. https://doi.org/10.1186/s13102-022-00468-4.

43. Schulze W, Richter J, Schulze B, Esenwein SA, Büttner-Janz K. Injury prophylaxis in paragliding. Br J Sports Med. 2002;36(5):365–9. https://doi.org/10.1136/bjsm.36.5.365.
44. Knapik JJ, Spiess A, Swedler DI, et al. Systematic review of the parachute ankle brace: injury risk reduction and cost effectiveness. Am J Prev Med. 2010;38:S182–8.
45. Knapik JJ, Darakjy S, Swedler D, Amoroso P, Jones BH. Parachute ankle brace and extrinsic injury risk factors during parachuting. Aviat Space Environ Med. 2008;79:408–15.
46. Søreide K. The epidemiology of injury in bungee jumping, BASE jumping, and skydiving. Med Sport Sci. 2012;58:112–29. https://doi.org/10.1159/000338720.
47. Jiang T, Tian S, Fan X, Chen T, Luo C, Yao J, Wang L. Kinematics and kinetics of lower-extremity joints in parachuting landing with backpack and knee brace. Med Eng Phys. 2020;86:1–7. https://doi.org/10.1016/j.medengphy.2020.10.009.
48. Feletti F, Aliverti A, Henjum M, Tarabini M, Brymer E. Incidents and injuries in foot-launched flying extreme sports. Aerosp Med Hum Perform. 2017;88(11):1016–23. https://doi.org/10.3357/AMHP.4745.2017.

MIX
Papier aus verantwortungsvollen Quellen
Paper from responsible sources
FSC® C105338

If you have any concerns about our products,
you can contact us on
ProductSafety@springernature.com

In case Publisher is established outside the EU,
the EU authorized representative is:
Springer Nature Customer Service Center GmbH
Europaplatz 3, 69115 Heidelberg, Germany

Printed by Libri Plureos GmbH
in Hamburg, Germany